Farewell
to Growth

— Farewell — to Growth

— Serge Latouche —

Translated by David Macey

polity

Ouvrage publié avec le concours du Ministère français de la Culture – Centre national du livre

Published with the assistance of the French Ministry of Culture – National Centre for the Book

First published in French as *Petit traité de la décroissance sereine* © Mille et une nuits, department de la Librairie Arthème Fayard, 2007

This English edition © Polity Press, 2009

Polity Press
65 Bridge Street
Cambridge CB2 1UR, UK

Polity Press
350 Main Street
Malden, MA 02148, USA

ISBN-13: 978-0-7456-4616-9
ISBN-13: 978-0-7456-4617-6(pb)

A catalogue record for this book is available from the British Library.

Typeset in 11 on 13 pt Sabon
by Toppan Best-set Premedia Limited
Printed and bound in Great Britain by MPG Books Limted, Bodmin, Cornwall

The publisher has used its best endeavours to ensure that the URLs for external websites referred to in this book are correct and active at the time of going to press. However, the publisher has no responsibility for the websites and can make no guarantee that a site will remain live or that the content is or will remain appropriate.

Every effort has been made to trace all copyright holders, but if any have been inadvertently overlooked the publishers will be pleased to include any necessary credits in any subsequent reprint or edition.

For further information on Polity, visit our website: www.politybooks.com

Contents

Preface

> If the fundamentalist belief in growth that rules the world
> today goes on like this, it will justify a naturalist
> fundamentalism that regards industry as evil.
>
> (Charbonneau 1981: 108)

In a kind review published in *Le Monde diplomatique* in
January 2005, Nicolas Truong described my previous
book (Latouche 2004a) as the 'breviary of the de-growth
[*décroissance*] movement'. His judgement was slightly
inaccurate in two respects: first, the project for a de-growth
society was no more than outlined in the conclusion, and,
second, a detailed analysis of what that project might
entail had yet to be made. De-growth was just one of the
avenues explored in *Survivre au développement*, the other
being 'localism'. What is more, the virtuous circle of convivial contraction, as described there, included only six
'R's, whereas it now includes eight.[1] Localism itself has
now been introduced and integrated into the circle in the

[1] It will be recalled that the eight independent objectives that can trigger
a virtuous circle of serene, convivial and sustainable contraction are:
re-evaluate, reconceptualize, restructure, redistribute, relocalize, reduce,
re-use and recycle.

form of 'relocalization' and 'reconceptualization'. And besides, that first outline had no suggestions to make about the political transition that would realize the utopia of de-growth in the North, and had nothing to say about the South. A more sophisticated project for an alternative society was outlined in *Le Pari de la décroissance* (Latouche 2006a), which the journal *L'Ecologiste* immediately described as the 'bible' of de-growth.[2]

And yet I went on playing with the idea of producing a short text that could bring together a summary of the corpus of the available analyses of de-growth. Whilst it synthesizes the main conclusions of *Le Pari de la décroissance* – and the reader who wishes to know more is invited to look at it – the present essay has its own contribution to make. It brings together recent developments in thinking about the subject, and especially the ideas that emerged during the debates that took place in the journal *Entropia*.[3] It is much more concerned with how the project can be concretely implemented at various levels. This book is therefore not so much 'Everything you always wanted to know about the subject but never dared ask', as a tool that can be used by anyone who is actively involved in environmental politics or political activist, especially at the local or regional level.

[2] *L'Ecologiste* no. 20, September–November 2006.
[3] 'Décroissance et politique', November 2006; 'Travail et décroissance', April 2007.

Introduction

If the earth must lose that great proportion of its
pleasantness which it owes to things that the unlimited
increase of wealth and population would extirpate from
it. . . . I sincerely hope, for the sake of posterity, that they
will be content to be stationary, long before necessity
compels them to it.

(Mill 2004 [1848]: 692)

There are, Woody Allen tells us, too many questions in
this world. Where do we come from? Where are we going?
And what are we going to eat tonight? For two-thirds of
humanity, the third question is still the most important,
but those of us who live in the North already consume too
much, and it is no longer a matter for concern. We consume
too much meat, too much fat, too much sugar and too
much salt. We are more likely to put on too much weight
than to go hungry. We run the risk of diabetes, cirrhosis
of the liver, cholesterol and obesity.[1] We would be healthier if we went on a diet. We have forgotten about the other

[1] Obesity affects 60% of the population of the United States, 30% of
that of Europe and 20% of children in France (Belpomme 2007: 138).

two questions but, although they are less urgent, they are still important. It will be recalled that the goals that the international 'community' set itself at the dawn of the third millennium included health for all and the eradication of poverty, and that those goals took priority over the fight against pollution. They were supposed to be achieved in 2015.

Where are we going? We are heading for a crash. We are in a performance car that has no driver, no reverse gear and no brakes and it is going to slam into the limitations of the planet.

We are in fact well aware of what is happening. Ever since Rachel Carson published *Silent Spring* in 1962, so many autonomous voices have spoken up that we cannot pretend that we do not know. The Club of Rome's famous report on *The Limits to Growth* (1972) warned us that the never-ending pursuit of growth was incompatible with the planet's' 'basics'.[2] New and damning reports are published every day, or almost every day. They are written from very different perspectives but they all confirm that common-sense diagnosis. The Wingspread Declaration (1991),[3] the Paris Memorandum of Appeal (2003)[4] and the Millennium Assessment Report,[5] were followed by reports from the Intergovernmental Experts' Report on

---

[2] The Club has since published *Beyond the Limits to Growth – An Update* (1992) and *Limits to Growth: The 30-Year Update* (2004). All three reports were produced under the editorship of Dennis Meadows.
[3] A statement by twenty-two biologists, most of them American, warning against the dangers of chemical products.
[4] An international declaration initiated by Professor Belpomme, alerting us to the health risks generated by economic growth.
[5] Millennium Assessment Reports on *Living beyond our Means: Natural Assets and Human Well-Being* (http:// www.millenniumassessement. org). This was a UN report based on the work of 1,360 specialists from 95 countries, published in Tokyo on 30 March 2005, demonstrating that human activity is abusing ecosystems' capacity for regeneration to such an extent as to compromise the economic, social and health objectives set by the international community for 2015.

climate change, from specialist NGOs (WWF, Greenpeace, Friends of the Earth, the Worldwatch Institute, etc.), semi-confidential reports from the Pentagon, and more confidential reports from the Bilderberg Foundation, Nicolas Stern's report to the British government, not to mention the appeals made by Jacques Chirac in Johannesburg, by Nicolas Hulot during the 2007 presidential campaign or by former American Vice-President Al Gore.

But we refuse to listen because we know where our next meal is coming from. And above all, we avoid the question of where we come from: from a growth society, or in other words a society that has been swallowed up by an economy whose only goal is growth for the sake of growth. It is significant that most *environmentalist* discourses make no critique of the growth society and confuse the issue with vague talk of sustainable development (see Hulot 2006). Denunciations of the 'frenzy of human activity' or of the enthusiasm for the word 'progress' are no substitute for an analysis of the capitalist and techno-economic marketing mega-machine. We are cogs in that machine, and we may well collude with it, but we are definitely not the driving force behind it. This system is based upon excess, and it is leading us into a blind alley. This schizophrenia puts theoreticians in a paradoxical position: they feel both that they are stating the obvious and that they are preaching in the wilderness. To say that exponential growth is incompatible with a finite world and that our capacity for consumption must not exceed the biosphere's capacity for regeneration is so obvious that few would disagree. It is, on the other hand, much more difficult to accept that the inevitable effects of production and consumption have to be reduced (by about two-thirds in the case of France) and that the logic of systematic and dramatic growth (which is driven by finance capital's compulsive addiction to growth) has to be called into question, as does our way of life. And as for naming those who are really responsible, that appears to be truly blasphemous.

Even though the stream is bursting its banks and threatens to wash everything away, we find it hard to accept the idea that we have to lower the water level, or in other words contract the economy. Yet we have to accept that idea if we are to emerge from the torpor that prevents us from taking action. We therefore have to (1) take stock of its implications; (2) offer an alternative to the insanity of the growth society in the form of the concrete utopia of de-growth; and (3) clarify how we can realize that utopia.

– 1 –

The Territory of De-Growth

Serious doubts then begin to arise in people's minds. Can
it be right to say that we have to produce too much so that
we can buy too much? That is the idea that dominates
the whole country's economic life. What will become of
us when the market is saturated and when we go on
producing? An advertising campaign has been launched to
persuade every family to buy two cars: one is not enough.
Can they be persuaded to buy three? We buy our cars, our
houses, our refrigerators, our overcoats and our shoes on
credit. But there will come a day when we have to settle
the bill.

> (Paul Hazard, *Le Malaise américain* [1931],
> cited Tertrais 2006: 66)

A UFO in the Microcosm of Politicking

Within the space of a few months, the theme of de-growth
made a remarkable breakthrough in both politics and the
media. It was for a long time a taboo subject, but it became
an object for debate for the Greens[1] (obviously), within

---

[1] See Latouche (2004e).

the Confédération paysanne[2] (which is not very surprising), in the so-called 'anti-globalization movement',[3] and even for a much wider public. It became an issue during the Italian national election campaign of 2006,[4] and then during the French presidential election of 2007.[5]

The idea is also central to the increasingly militant protests, at both the regional and local levels, against '*les grands projets*'. The resistance is spreading in Italy, with protests in the Susa valley, against the Lyon–Turin high-speed train and its monstrous tunnel, against the mega-bridge over the Straits of Messina, against the Moses project to use mobile flood barriers to protect the Venice lagoon, against incinerators (in Trento and elsewhere) and against the coal-fired nuclear power station in Citavecchia, and so on. In France, opposition to the *grands projets*, coal-fired power stations, the Iter (International Thermonuclear Experimental Reactor) project and big infrastructural transport projects is less coordinated and less developed because of French centralization and the power of the administration, but it is beginning to spread.[6]

All over France and Italy, and more recently Belgium and Spain, de-growth groups are spontaneously emerging,

---

[2] See Latouche (2004c). The Confédération paysanne was founded in 1987 when two smaller unions merged. A member of the Via Campesina, it supports and encourages an environmentally friendly 'peasant agriculture' (Translator).

[3] See the dossier on de-growth, *Politis*, 11 December 2003.

[4] The idea was taken up by the Italian Greens (I Verdi) but led to friction between Rifondazione and the other parties in the anti-Berlusconi coalition. Paulo Cacciari, who was Rifondazione's candidate, was elected to represent Venice after having published a plea for economic contraction (see Cacciari 2006). Maurizio Pallante, who wrote the manifesto *La Decrescita felice* (Pallante 2005), was an adviser to the Green Minister for the Environment following the 2006 elections.

[5] It had the explicit support of the Greens' Yves Cochet, and the rather less explicit support of José Bové. All the presidential candidates faced questions about the issue.

[6] See Charbonneau (n.d.), Jean Monestier (2007a) and 'La Grande Illusion des aéroports régionaux', *Fil du Conflent* 14, April–May 2007.

organizing marches and establishing networks. The de-growth approach is inspiring both individual and collective action. Examples include the Cambiaresti movement, which is trying to promote a 'just balance sheet', or in other words a fair ecological footprint (1,300 families in Venetia alone), AMAP in France (Associations pour le Maintien d'une Agriculture Paysanne), the GAS (Groupe d'acheteurs solidaires; 'purchasers' solidarity group') in France, and the advocates of voluntary simplicity in Italy (Martin 2007; see also Latouche 2006a: 101–11). The emergence of this movement, which is a UFO in the microcosm of politicking, caused a great stir in the media. Newspapers, the radio and even television became involved. Whilst some of the media tried to provide serious information,[7] others decided for or against without taking the trouble to find out what was at stake, and usually distorted the few analyses that were available. What is behind this 'new concept' of de-growth? Is it soluble in sustainable development? Where does the concept come from? Do we need it? These are the questions that usually arise time after time.

What is De-Growth?

'De-growth' is a political slogan with theoretical implications, or what Paul Ariès (2005) calls an 'explosive word' that is designed to silence the chatter of those who are addicted to productivism. Given that the opposite of a perverse idea does not necessarily give rise to a virtuous idea, I am not recommending de-growth for the sake of de-growth. That would be absurd, but, all things considered, no more absurd than preaching the gospel of growth for the sake of growth. The slogan of 'de-growth'

[7] We could cite *Politis*, *Carta*, *Le Monde diplomatique*, the journal *La Décroissance*, its Italian equivalent *La decrescita* and *Entropia*, which was mentioned above.

is primarily designed to make it perfectly clear that we must abandon the goal of exponential growth, as that goal is promoted by nothing other than a quest for profits on the part of the owners of capital and has disastrous implications for the environment, and therefore for humanity. It is not just that society is reduced to being nothing more than an instrument or a means to be used by the productive mechanism; human beings themselves are becoming the waste products of a system that would like to make them useless and do without them.[8]

De-growth is not, in my view, the same thing as negative growth. That expression is an absurd oxymoron, but it is a clear indication of the extent to which we are dominated by the imaginary of growth.[9] We know that simply contracting the economy plunges our societies into disarray, increases the rate of unemployment and hastens the demise of the health, social, educational, cultural and environmental projects that provide us with an indispensable minimal quality of life. It is not difficult to imagine the catastrophes that negative growth would bring about! Just as there is nothing worse than a work-based society in which there is no work, there is nothing worse than a growth-based society in which growth does not materialize. And that social and civilizational regression is precisely what is in store for us if we do not change direction. For all these reasons, de-growth is conceivable only in a de-growth society, or in other words within the framework of a system that is based upon a different logic. The alternative really is: de-growth or barbarism.

Strictly speaking, we should be talking at the theoretical level of 'a-growth', in the sense in which we speak of 'a-theism', rather than 'de-growth'. And we do indeed have to abandon a faith or a religion – that of the economy, progress and development – and reject the irrational and quasi-idolatrous cult of growth for growth's sake.

---

[8] 'The idea that economic growth is an end in itself implies that society is a means' (Flahaut 2005: 6).
[9] Its literal meaning appears to be 'advance by going backwards'.

To begin with, 'de-growth' is therefore no more than a banner that can rally those who have made a radical critique of development (see Latouche 2001), and who want to outline the contours of an alternative project for a post-development politics.[10] Its goal is to build a society in which we can live better lives whilst working less and consuming less.[11] It is an essential proposition if we are to open up a space for the inventiveness and creativity of the imagination, which has been blocked by economistic, developmentalist and progressive totalitarianism.

The Battle over Words and Ideas

Attempts are often made to subsume de-growth under the rubric of sustainable development, presumably so as to neutralize its subversive potential, even though the term has to be used if we are to get away from the posturing and confusion created by a 'catch-all' term that we even find plastered on packets of Lavazza coffee. Further evidence that sustainable development is, like so many other things, a mystification is supplied by statements from captains of industry like Nestlé's director general ('Sustainable development is easily defined: if your great-grandfather, your grandfather and your children remain loyal

---

[10] See 'Brouillons pour l'avenir: contributions au débat sur les alternatives', *Les Nouveaux Cahiers de l'UED*, 14, Paris and Geneva: PUF, 2003.
[11] This corresponds quite closely to what André Gorz (1994 [1991]: 33–4]) used to call 'ecological rationalization' (a somewhat unfortunate term): ' "Ecological rationalization" can be summed up in the slogan "less but better". . . . Ecological modernization requires that investment no longer serve the growth of the economy but its contraction – that is to say, it requires the sphere governed by economic rationality in the modern sense to shrink. There can be no ecological modernization without restricting the dynamic of capitalist accumulation and reducing consumption by self-imposed restraint. The exigencies of ecological modernization coincide with those of a transformed North–South relationship, and with the original aims of socialism.'

customers of Nestlé, then we have been working in a sustainable way. And five million people around the world are loyal Nestlé customers'[12]) or the supermarket-owner Michel-Édouard Leclerc ('The term [sustainable development] is so broad that it can be applied to anything and everything. We can all claim to be practising sustainable development in the same way that Molière's Monsieur Jourdain spoke prose without realizing it. It is also true to say that it's a fashionable *concept*. Both in the world of business and in any social debate. So what? Shopkeepers have always been good at recuperating good slogans').[13]

We can all agree that the expression is at once a pleonasm at the definitional level and an oxymoron at the level of its content. It is a pleonasm because, according to Rostow, development means 'self-sustaining growth'. And it is an oxymoron because development is neither sustainable nor self-sustaining.[14]

Let us be quite clear about this: the problem has little to do with 'sustainability', which is in some sense related to the philosopher Hans Jonas's 'imperative of responsibility' (Jonas 1984 [1979]). That imperative is cheerfully ignored by development actors such as the nuclear industry, genetically modified (GM) crops, mobile phones, pesticides and the REACH directive.[15] Without going back to the emblematic case of asbestosis, the list of areas where it is not applied is endless. The word 'development' is

---

[12] Peter Brabeck-Letmathe, director general of Nestlé, addressing the 2003 Davos forum, cited Jacquiau (2006: 151).

[13] Michel-Edouard Leclerc in *Le Nouvel Economiste*, 26 March 2004, cited Jacquiau (2006: 281).

[14] It is interesting to note that, according to the WWF's report for 2006, only one country meets the criteria for sustainable development, namely a high level of human development and a sustainable ecological footprint. That country is Cuba. Despite that, and despite all the data it supplies, the Stern report puts an optimistic face on things (as does Nicolas Hulot) and claims: 'We can be green and grow.'

[15] The acronym REACH stands for Registration, Evaluation, Authorization and Restriction of Chemicals.

toxic, no matter which adjective we use to dress it up.[16] Sustainable development has now found the perfect way to square the circle: 'clean development mechanisms'. The expression refers to technologies that save energy or carbon and that are described as being eco-efficient. This is more verbal diplomacy. The undeniable and desirable advances that have been made in technology do nothing to challenge to the suicidal logic of development. This is another way of patching things up so as to avoid having to change them.

The class struggle and political battles go on in the arena of words too. We know that we were seduced into accepting an ethnocentric and ethnocidal concept of development, but it went hand in hand with the violence of colonization and imperialism, and represents what Aminata Traoré eloquently describes as a real 'rape of the imaginary' (Traoré 2002).

The battle of words is raging, even when it is just a matter of introducing what appear to be very minor semantic nuances. Towards the end of the 1970s, for instance, the expression 'sustainable development' appeared to triumph over the more neutral 'eco-development', which was adopted at the 1972 Stockholm Conference as a result of the pressures brought to bear by the American industrial lobby and thanks to the personal intervention of Henry Kissinger.

It is quite obvious that these quibbles mask differences of opinion, different worldviews, and different interests (and they are not just intellectual interests).[17] Hervé Kempf

---

[16] Even a conventional economist like Claudio Napoleoni could write towards the end of his life: 'We cannot just go on dreaming up "new models for development". The expression "new model for development" is meaningless. . . . I do not believe that we can simultaneously solve the problem of stronger growth and that of qualitative changes in development' (1990: 92).

[17] The 'alternative' movement is no exception. 'I fought against the word "growth", which was usurping the word "development", states Alain Lipietz (2006: 117), 'And I am now fighting the word 'de-growth".'

(2007) makes it clear that the sole function of the 'sustainable development' that is ritually invoked in all political programmes is to 'maintain levels of profit and to avoid changing our habits by making an imperceptible change of direction'.[18] Talk of 'different' development or 'different' growth is either very naïve or quite duplicitous. For the record, it should be recalled that when the Chair of the European Commission Sicco Mansholt, having learned the lessons of the Club of Rome's first report, was so bold as to try to steer Brussels' policies in a direction that might challenge the need for growth, the French Commissioner Raymond Barre disagreed with him in public. It was finally agreed that growth should be made more human and fairer. Well, it was a start. We know what happened next. At the time, the Secretary General of the French Communist Party denounced the 'monstrous programme' of the leaders of the European Economic Community (EEC). Things have changed for the better. According to the Confédération Générale du Travail's Bernard Saincy, a new phase began in 2006, when the CGT adopted a programme of sustainable development and used the phrase 'giving growth a new content'.[19] One more effort, comrades!

We certainly have to make a distinction between 'development' and 'growth' (both lower case), which are evolutionary phenomena affecting specific realities (population, potato production, quantities of waste, toxicity of water, etc.), and Development and Growth (upper case), which are abstract concepts referring to an economic dynamism that is an end in itself. It is not our fault if the two get confused; the confusion is deliberately sustained by the dominant ideology.

[18] He then adds: 'But it is profits and habits that prevent us from changing direction.'
[19] Bernard Saincy interviewed by Fabrice Flipo, 'CGT et Amis de la Terre: quels compromis possibles?' *Cosmopolitiques*, no. 13: 176.

And yet, if the other world we want so much is not to look too much like the world we live in, it is high time we decolonized our imaginaries. It is by no means certain that we have another thirty years to do so.

The Two Sources of De-Growth

Whilst the term 'de-growth' is a very recent addition to economic, political and social debates, the ideas it conveys have a much longer history and are bound up with both *culturalist* and ecological critiques of economics. The 'thermo-industrial' society caused so much suffering and so many injustices that many thought it undesirable from the outset. Whilst industrialization and technology have, if we ignore the Luddite phase,[20] come in for little criticism until recent times, all the human sciences have denounced *homo economicus*, who provides the anthropological basis for both the theory and the practice of economics, as reductive (see Latouche 2005a). Both the theoretical basis and practical implementation (modern society) of economics have been called into question by the sociology of Émile Durkheim and Marcel Mauss, the anthropology of Karl Polanyi and Marshall Sahlins, and by the psychoanalysis of Erich Fromm and Gregory Bateson. The project for an autonomous and economical society is not a recent invention. Without going back to the utopias of the early socialists[21] or to the anarchist tradition that was revitalized by situationism, such projects were being drawn up from the 1960s onwards, and in forms very similar to those outlined here, by André Gorz, François Partant, Jacques Ellul

---

[20] A British labour movement of the period 1811–12, named after its leader Ned Ludd and famous for its destruction of machines (power looms).
[21] Even though some of them were, as Thierry Paquot (2007b) reminds us, genuine precursors of de-growth.

and Bernard Charbonneau, and especially by Cornelius Castoriadis and Ivan Illich.[22] The failure of development in the South and the loss of any sense of direction in the North led these thinkers to call into question the consumer society and its imaginary bases, namely progress, science and technology.

This critique led to the search for a 'post-development'. At the same time, a growing awareness of the ecological crisis introduced a new dimension: the growth society was not just undesirable but also unsustainable!

The intuitive realization that there are physical limits to economic growth probably goes back to Malthus (1766–1834), but it was only with Sidi Carnot and his second law of thermodynamics (1824) that it acquired a scientific basis. The fact that transformations of energy (into different forms such as heat, motion, etc.) cannot be totally reversed – and that we come up against the phenomenon of entropy – could not fail to have implications for an economy based on those very transformations. If we turn to those who pioneered the application of the laws of thermodynamics to economics, special mention should be made of Sergei Podolinsky, who was the architect of an energy-based economics that tried to reconcile socialism with ecology.[23] It was, however, only in the 1970s that the question of ecology became a central issue for economics, thanks mainly to the work of the great Romanian scientist and economist Nicholas Georgescu-Roegen (1971), who saw that the law of entropy had bio-economic implications, as Alfred Lotka, Erwin Schrödinger, Norbert Wiener and Léon Brillouin had already sensed in the 1940s and 1950s.[24] When it adapted the model of classical

---

[22] Mention should, perhaps, also be made of the great American philosopher John Dewey, who was Henry David Thoreau's disciple. See the analysis made by Philippe Chanial (2006).

[23] Sergei Podolisky (1850–1891): Ukrainian aristocrat exiled in Paris who tried unsuccessfully to interest Marx in the ecological critique.

[24] For a short history of de-growth, see Grinevald (2006).

Newtonian mechanics, notes Georgescu-Roegen, economics forgot that time is irreversible. It therefore overlooked
entropy, or in other words the non-reversibility of transformations of energy and matter. Waste and pollution are,
for instance, products of economic activity, but they are
not functions of standard production.

The last link with nature was broken when the earth
ceased to be seen as a function of standard production
in about 1880. Now that there was no longer any reference to any biophysical substratum, there appeared to be
no ecological limits to economic production, as conceived
by most neo-classical theorists. What were the implications of this? The unthinking waste of available but scarce
resources, and under-use of abundant supplies of solar
energy. As Yves Cochet notes (2005: 147), 'the mathe-
matical elegance of contemporary neoclassical economic
theory masks its indifference to the basic laws of biology,
chemistry and physics, and especially the laws of thermodynamics.' It is ecological nonsense.[25] The real economic process, unlike the theoretical model, is not, in
short, a purely mechanical and reversible process; it is by
its very nature *entropic* and takes place in a biosphere
that functions within a temporality that is not reversible.[26]
Hence, according to Georgescu-Roegen, the impossibility
of infinite growth in a finite world, and hence the need
to replace traditional economic science with a *bioeconom-
ics*, or in other words the need to relate economics to
the biosphere. The term *décroissance* (in French) is used
as the title of a collection of his essays (Georgescu-Roegen
1994).

Kenneth Boulding is one of the few economists to
have seen the implications of this. In an article published

---

[25] 'One nugget of pure gold contains more energy than the same number
of atoms dissolved one at a time in sea water' (Cochet 2005: 153).
[26] He also writes (1994: 63): 'We cannot produce bigger and better
refrigerators, cars or jet planes without producing bigger and better
waste.'

in 1966, he contrasts the 'cowboy economy', in which
the maximization of consumption is based upon predation and the pillaging of natural resources, with the
'spaceman economy', 'in which the earth has become
a single spaceship, without unlimited reservoirs of
anything, either for extraction or pollution' (Boulding
1996 [1966]: 362, cited Clerc 2006: 17). He concludes
that anyone who believes that exponential growth can go
on for ever in a finite world is either a madman or an
economist.

Addiction to Growth

> All the activity of shopkeepers and advertising executives
> consists in creating needs in a world that is collapsing
> under the weight of production. This requires an
> increasingly rapid rotation and consumption of products,
> and therefore the production of more and more waste.
> Waste-disposal is an increasingly important business.
>
> (Maris 2006: 49)

Our society's fate is tied up with an organization that is
based upon endless accumulation. That system is condemned to grow. As soon as growth slows down or comes
to a halt, there is a crisis, or even panic. We are back to
old Marx's 'Accumulate, accumulate! That is the law and
the prophets!' The need to accumulate means that growth
is an 'iron corset'. Jobs, retirement pensions and increased
public spending (education, law and order, justice, culture,
transport, health, etc.) all presuppose a constant rise in
Gross Domestic Product (GDP). 'The only antidote to
permanent unemployment is growth,' insists Nicolas
Baverez (2003), a 'declinologist' who is close to Sarkozy,
and many in the anti-globalization movement agree with
him. Ultimately, the virtuous circle becomes a hellish circle.
The life of a worker usually comes down to that of a 'bio-

ingester who uses commodities to metabolize his wages and his wages to metabolize commodities as he goes from the factory to the hypermarket and from the hypermarket to the factory' (Cacciari 2006: 102).

Three ingredients are necessary if the consumer society is to go on with the merry dance that is taking it to hell: advertising, which creates the desire to consume; credit, which gives us the means to consume; and products with built-in and or planned obsolescence, which means that we always need new products. The three mainsprings behind the consumer society really do drive people to crime.

Advertising makes us want what we do not have and despise what we already have. It creates and re-creates the dissatisfaction and tension of frustrated desire. When the presidents of big American companies were surveyed, 90% of them admitted that it would be impossible to sell a new product without an advertising campaign; 85% stated that advertising 'often' persuaded people to buy things they did not need; and 51% said that advertising persuaded people to buy things that they did not really want (Gorz 1994 [1991]). Prime necessities have been forgotten. Increasingly, demand no longer centres on very useful goods, but on very useless goods (Cacciari 2006: 29). Advertising is an essential element in the vicious and suicidal circle of exponential growth. It is now the second biggest budget in the world, after arms, and is incredibly greedy: 103 billion euros in the United States in 2003, and 15 billion in France. In 2004, French companies invested 31.2 billion euros in communications (equivalent to 2% of GDP, and twice the French Social Security deficit). In all, the world spends over 500 billion euros on advertising every year. That is a colossal amount of material, visual, audio, mental and spiritual pollution. The advertising system has 'taken over the streets, invaded – and disfigured – collective space, and is appropriating everything that is meant to be public: roads, towns, means of transport, stations, sports grounds,

beaches and festivals' (Besset 2005: 251).[27] Television programmes are interrupted by advertising breaks, children
are being manipulated and upset (because the weakest are
in the front line) and forests are being destroyed (we get
40 kg of paper through our letter boxes every year). And
ultimately, it is consumers who pick up the bill to the tune
of 500 euros per year per person.

  For its part, the use of cash and credit, which are essential if those on inadequate incomes are to consume and if
businesspeople are to invest without having the capital
they need to do so, is a powerful 'dictator' of growth in
the North but also has much more destructive and tragic
effects in the South.[28] The 'diabolical' logic of money that
always demands more money is none other than the logic
of capital. We are faced with what Georgio Ruffolo (2006)
nicely terms the 'terrorism of compound interest'. No
matter what we call it in an attempt to legitimate it –
return on equity, shareholder value – and no matter
whether we obtain it by cost killing, downsizing, extorting
abusive property legislation (patents on living matter) or
establishing a monopoly (Microsoft), we are still talking
about profit, which is the motor behind the market
economy and capitalism, whatever mutations they might
undergo. The quest for profit at any cost is pursued by
expanding production–consumption and cutting costs.

---

[27] The author adds: 'It is flooding our nights in the same way that it is
taking over our days, cannibalizing the Internet, colonizing the newspapers, making some of them financially dependent on it and reducing
others to pitiful platforms for adverts. Television is its weapon of mass
destruction, and it has established a dictatorship of the ratings over the
main cultural vector of our times. That is not enough. Advertising is
also making an assault on private life, letter boxes, messaging services,
telephones, video games and the radios in our bathrooms. And it is now
taking over the grapevine. . . . We are being attacked from all sides and
there is no let-up. Mental pollution, visual pollution, noise pollution.'
[28] According to the Federal Bank, household debt in America reached
the astronomical level of $28.189 million in 2007. That represents
248% of GDP.

The new heroes of the day are the cost killers, or the managers whom transnational companies fight to recruit by offering them stock options and golden parachutes. Mostly the products of business schools, which might be more accurately described as 'schools of economic warfare', these strategists are intent on doing all they can to outsource costs, which are borne by their employees, their sub-contracts, the countries of the South, their clients, states and public services, future generations and, above all, nature, which has become both a supplier of resources and a dustbin. All capitalists and financiers, as well as any *homo economicus* (meaning all of us), tend to become ordinary 'criminals' who collude to some extent in the economic banality of evil (see Latouche 2003a).

The American market analyst Victor Lebow understood the logic of consumerism as early as the 1950s. Writing in the *Journal of Retailing* (Lebow 1955: 7), he notes that 'Our enormously productive economy demands that we make consumption our way of life, that we convert the buying and use of goods into rituals, that we seek our spiritual satisfaction, our ego satisfaction, in consumption. . . . We need things consumed, burned up, replaced and discarded at an ever-accelerating rate.' Built-in obsolescence gives the growth society the ultimate weapon of consumerism. Appliances and equipment, from electric lamps to spectacles, break more and more quickly because some part is designed to fail. It is impossible to find spares, or someone to repair them. And even if we could lay hands on someone who could repair them, it would be cheaper to buy new ones (and they are now manufactured at knockdown prices in the sweatshops of South-East Asia). That is why mountains of computers, televisions, refrigerators, dish-washers, DVD players and mobile phones fill up our tips and dustbins, and increase the risk of pollution. Every year, 150 million computers are shipped to the Third World for sorting and recycling (500 ships sail for Nigeria every month), and they contain toxic heavy metals such as mercury, nickel, cadmium, arsenic and lead (Gras 2006).

We have become addicted to the drug of growth. 'Toxic addiction to growth' is not, as it happens, a metaphor. It is polymorphous. The consumerist bulimia of those who are addicted to supermarkets and department stores is no different from the workaholism of managers, whose addiction is further stimulated, if need be, by over-consumption of anti-depressants and, according to British studies, the use of cocaine by senior managers who want to be 'up to it'. The hyper-consumption of the contemporary individual, who has become a 'turbo-consumer', leads to a damaged or paradoxical happiness (Lipovetsky 2006). Never before have human beings been in such a state of dereliction. The 'consolation goods' industry tries in vain to compensate for it (see Leclair 1998). Sadly, the French are the record-holders: in 2005, we bought 41 million boxes of anti-depressants (Canfin 2006). Without going into details about these 'human-generated illnesses', we can only confirm Professor Belpomme's diagnosis: 'Growth has become humanity's cancer' (Belpomme 2007).

The Green Algae and the Snail

Do we really believe that exponential growth can go on for ever in a finite world? Our earth is – fortunately – certainly not a closed system. It receives energy from the sun, and cannot do without it. Yet even if much better use were made of that energy, the quantity of energy it receives is limited and does nothing to change its available surface area or its stock of rare materials. And yet there are economists who claim that 'so long as the sun goes on shining, there are no unavoidable "scientific" limits to the development of economic activity on earth, apart from, naturally, the ecological disasters that might potentially be triggered by human activity itself.' They therefore conclude that 'Our only chance of correcting [these dysfunctionalities] in time is to make even more progress towards understanding and mastering our environment. And therefore to make the world even more artificial' (Duval 2006: 38, 41). So the only way we can enjoy the luxury of de-growth is to go on growing, so to speak.[29]

The ancient wisdom of living in harmony with an environment that we exploit in reasonable ways has given way to *hubris*, or the overweening pride of the masters and possessors of nature. This quantitative madness will inevitably make our lives unbearable because of the 'terrorism of compound interest'. This is what might be called the green algae theorem, which is a variation on Albert Jacquart's water lily paradox (Jacquart 1998).

Encouraged by the local farmers' excessive use of chemical fertilizers, a bloom of green algae set up home in a very big pond one day. Although its annual growth rate was rapid – it doubled in size every year – no one was worried. Even if it did double in size every year, only 3% of the pond's surface would be covered in twenty-four years. People did begin to get a little worried when it had colonized half the surface. At that point, eutrophication became a distinct possibility: sub-aquatic life might be asphyxiated. The problem was that, although it had taken several decades to reach this point, it would now take only one year for the lake's ecosystem to die completely.

We have now reached the point where the green algae bloom has colonized half the pond. If we do not act very quickly and very effectively, we will soon die of asphyxiation. Because we in the West have embraced the logic of geometric progression that governs economic growth, we have abandoned the attempt to control it. If per capita GDP continues to grow by 3.5% per year (and this was France's average rate of growth from 1949 to 1959), it will have grown by a multiple of 31 in a century, and by 961 in two hundred years. An annual growth rate of 10%,

[29] For a refutation of this fantasy, which has no material basis, see Latouche (2006a).

as in China today, will increase by a multiple of 736 in one hundred years (Jouvenel 2002 [1968]). A 3% rate of growth multiplies GDP by 20 in one hundred years, by 40 in two hundred years, and by 8,000 in three hundred years. If growth automatically generated well-being, we would now be living in paradise. We are in fact going down the road to hell.

In these conditions, rediscovering the wisdom of the snail is a matter of urgency. The snail teaches us the need to move slowly, but it also teaches us an even more important lesson:

> A snail, after adding a number of widening rings to the delicate structure of its shell, suddenly brings its accustomed activities to a stop. A single additional ring would increase the size of the shell sixteen times. Instead of contributing to the welfare of the snail, it would burden the creature with such an excess of weight that any increase in its productivity would henceforth be literally outweighed by the task of coping with the difficulties created by enlarging the shell beyond the limits set by its purpose. At that point, the problems of overgrowth begin to multiply geometrically, while the snail's biological capacity can be best extended arithmetically. (Illich 1983: 82)

The snail's abandonment of geometrical reason, which it, too, adopted for a while, points the way to a 'de-growth' society, and perhaps a serene and convivial society.[30]

---

[30] Geometrical reason can, in theory, be used in a different way. 'An annual de-growth rate of 1% saves 25% (of output) in 29 years, and 50% in 69 years. An annual de-growth rate of 2% saves 50% in 34 years, 64% in 50 years, and 87% in 100 years' (Ariès 2005: 90). The main point of this argument is of course that it is a theoretical refutation of our opponents, who accuse us of wanting to take them back to the Stone Age. De-growth is definitely not the exact opposite of growth; it is a way of building an autonomous society. Such a society would certainly be more sober; what is more important, it would also be more balanced.

An Unsustainable Ecological Footprint

Our economic *hypergrowth* is coming up against the limits of the biosphere's finite resources. The earth's capacity for regeneration can no longer keep up with demand: human beings are turning resources into waste faster than nature can transform waste into new resources (WWF 2006: 1). If we measure the environmental impact of our way of life in terms of the ecological 'footprint' it leaves on the surface of the earth or on the bioproductive space we need, the results are unsustainable both in terms of the fairness of our right to draw on nature and in terms of the biosphere's carrying capacity. There are limits to the space that is available to us on Planet Earth. It represents 51 million hectares. 'Bioproductive' space, or the space we can use to reproduce ourselves, is a mere fraction of the whole: some 12 billion hectares.[31] If we divide that figure by the present population of the world, we have approximately 1.8 hectares per person. If we take into account the need for energy and raw materials, the surface area required to absorb the waste and reject produced by production and consumption (every time we burn a litre of oil, it takes one year for five square metres of forest to absorb the CO_2!), and then factor in the impact of the necessary habitat and infrastructures, researchers at California's Redefining Progress and the World Wild Foundation (WWF) calculate that every individual consumes an average of 2.2 hectares of bioproductive space – assuming that the population remains stable. We are already living on credit. What is more, this average footprint conceals some very big disparities. A citizen of the United States consumes 9.6 hectares, a Canadian 7.2, a European 4.5, a French citizen 5.26, and an Italian 3.8. Even though there are significant

---

[31] One hectare of permanent grazing land is considered to be equivalent to 0.48 hectares of bioproductive space; the equivalent ratio for a fishing zone is 0.36 (Wackernagel 2005).

differences in the available amount of bioproductive space in different countries, this is a very long way from global equality (Cacciari 2006: 27).[32] Humanity is, in other words, already consuming almost 30% of the biosphere's capacity for regeneration. If everyone had the same life style as the French, we would need three planets; if we all followed the example of our friends in America, we would need six.

How is this possible? Two phenomena make it possible. First, we are like spendthrift children and, being unable to live on our income, we are spending our inheritance. In the space of a few decades, we have burned what it took the planet millions of years to produce. Our annual consumption of coal and oil is equivalent to a biomass accumulated beneath the crust of the earth over a period of 100,000 years of photosynthesis.[33] Those of who live in the North also receive massive technical aid from the countries of the South. Most countries in Africa consume less than 0.2 hectares of bioproductive space, but they provide us with fodder for our livestock. One hectare of woodland has to be destroyed to produce one tonne of soy cattle-cake. If we have not changed direction by 2050, the ecological debt, or in other words the cumulative deficit, will be equivalent to thirty-four years of biological productivity on the part of the entire planet (WWF 2006: 22). Even if Africans tightened their belts still further, we do not have the thirty-four planets it would take to reimburse them.

---

[32] Cf. Cochet and Sinaï (2003: 38): 'The total per capita need for raw materials in the United States is currently 80 tonnes per annum. But . . . it takes some 300 kg of raw materials to generate an income of $100.'

[33] According to the calculations of the German historian R. Peter Sieferle (in Bevilacqua 2001: 112). One litre of petrol is the product of 23 tonnes of organic matter transformed over a period of one million years (Belpomme 2007: 229).

Our system went into the wrong orbit in the eighteenth century, but the ecological debt is a recent phenomenon. At the global level, it rose from 70% of the planet in 1960 to 120% in 1999.[34]

If biodiversity is to be preserved, it is also essential to save part of the biosphere's productive capacity in order to guarantee the survival of other species, and especially wild species. These biosphere reserves must be distributed equally across different biogeographic zones and the major biomes (WWF 2006: 3). It is estimated that the minimal threshold that must be preserved represents 10% of bioproductive space,[35] and it would be not unreasonable to introduce a moratorium in order to ensure that is still available for the animal and plant species in question.

A False Solution: Reducing the Population

Can't the equation of ecological sustainability be solved by reducing the size of the denominator until we get back to the right footprint? Conservative politicians do recommend this lazy solution. On 10 December 1974 Henry Kissinger published his National State Security Memorandum 200 on 'Implications of Worldwide Population Growth for US Security and Overseas Interests'.[36] It suggested that the population of thirteen Third World

---

[34] 'Humanity's grazing footprint rose by 80% between 1961 and 1999' (Cochet and Sinaï 2003: 36).
[35] According to Jean-Paul Besset (2005: 318), 'Sharing space with other species and leaving them, for example, 20% of the space on earth that humanity has not already appropriated implies interrupting the systematic character of the process of development, infrastructure and urbanization.'
[36] The full text of NSSM 200 is reprinted in Mumford (1996: 435–558).

countries (India, Bangladesh, Nigeria) had to be contained, if not reduced, to perpetuate America's global hegemony and to guarantee Americans access to strategic minerals all over the world. The demographic weight of those countries alone meant that they were, so to speak, destined to play a major role in internal politics. In order to achieve that goal, Third World leaders were to be given incentives to persuade them to accept birth control methods (whilst taking care to ensure that such pressure did not look like a form of economic or racial American imperialism). And if that plan were to fail, it might be necessary to resort to more coercive methods. Public health specialist Maurice H. King shared the same view, and argued that if family planning did not work, the poor should be left to die because they posed an ecological threat (cited Tertrais 2006: 35). The American author William Vogt was already recommending drastic population cuts in the 1950s and suggesting that a large-scale bacteriological war would, if waged energetically, be an effective way of giving the earth its forests and grazing lands back (Tertrais 2006: 35). The notion that reducing the population is the 'final solution' to the ecological problem is based on a number of common-sense truisms, such as a finite planet is incompatible with an infinite population.

According to David Lord-Nicholson (2006: 20), who shares this view,

> The truth is that greener lifestyles can make a difference but that zero-impact living, for the foreseeable future, is a chimera and that human numbers do matter, hugely. Footprinting studies by Andrew Ferguson at the Optimum Population Trust suggest that if a world of six billion lived a 'modest' western European lifestyle based entirely on renewable energy, it would still need, to support it, another 1.8 planets.

François Meyer sounded the alarm bell in the 1970s with his *La Surchauffe de la croissance* (Meyer 1974). According to Meyer, a hyper-exponential rate of demographic growth is a major phenomenon that is taking us further and further away from any logistical solution that might restore a certain equilibrium.[37] Assuming that there are 135 million km[2] of land above water level, he calculates that in 1650, the surface area theoretically available per individual was 0.28 km[2]; in 1970, it was no more than 0.04 km[2], or seven times less. By 2070, it will in all probability be reduced to 0.011 km[2], or four times less, and that does not leave us enough bioproductive space to survive.

The converse view is just as mechanical, but it is optimistic: in the time that it took the world's population to rise by a coefficient of 6, leading to an increase from 1 to 6 billion over a period of two hundred years, the productive forces increased several hundred times. There is therefore no cause for concern.

How many of us will there be in 2050? That is the symbolic (and arbitrary) date of the moment of truth when the effects of climate change, the exhaustion of oil reserves (and even fish stocks[38]) and of foreseeable economic and financial crises will all converge. Thirty-five years ago, the Club of Rome's first report predicted that there would be between 12 and 15 million of us. Demographers using the demographic 'transition' model suggest a figure of 9 billion. There will be many fewer of us if the sterilization of the species continues as a result of the ingestion of reprotoxic substances: humanity may be heading for extinction. It is difficult to prophesy what will happen. According to Professor Belpomme (2007: 194),

---

[37] See also Meyer (1954). Albert Jacquart (1998) also notes that, given a constant annual growth rate of 0.5%, the human population, which numbered about 250 million individuals at the beginning of our era, would be about 5,000 billion today.

[38] According to an FAO report (Worm et al. 2006), the oceans and all fish stocks will be exhausted by 2048 if fishing continues at the current rate.

Five scenarios might result in our extinction: suicide through violence, such as a nuclear war . . . the emergence of extremely serious illness, such as an infectious pandemic or sterility leading to an irreversible demographic decline, the exhaustion of natural resources . . . the destruction of biodiversity . . . extreme physical-chemical transformations of our inner environment, such as the loss of the ozone layer or worsening of the greenhouse effect.

These approaches avoid, however, the real problem of the logic of excess that governs our economic system. Once we have dealt with that and made the paradigm shift we need to make, the demographic issue can be approached and resolved more calmly. The constraints are elastic. Over-consumption of meat on the part of the rich, which is the source of many health and ecological problems, means that 35% of the planet's arable land (in addition to the 30% of natural grazing land above water level [Paquot 2007a: 13]) has to be given over to the production of animal fodder. A relative cut in stock breeding and improved treatment of livestock would allow us both to feed a larger population better and to cut carbon dioxide emissions.[39] We can agree with Jean-Pierre Tertrais (2006: 37) that

> There is little point in speculating about the mathematical aspects of variations in the human species: population levels have to be stabilized this century. The central issue is whether that will result from events, authoritarian policies or even methods based upon coercion or even barbarism, or whether it will be the result of a deliberate choice and a refusal to allow the desire to procreate to be programmed by a so-called enlightened elite.

[39] It should be recalled that the livestock industry is responsible for 37% of the methane emissions that result from human activity, or in other words an amount equivalent to more than the CO_2 emissions produced by the transport sector.

Perhaps the last word should be left to someone with a specialist knowledge of our wise cousins the bonobos: 'The question facing a growing world population is not as much whether or not we can handle crowding, but if we will be fair and just in the distribution of resources' (Waal 2005: 168). That is the challenge laid down by de-growth.

The Political Corruption of Growth

During the *trente glorieuses*, we could denounce the harmful effects of growth and development in the South. That is where they were most obvious because they resulted in deculturation, homoegenization and pauperization. Whilst pauperization in the economic sense seemed counter-intuitive in the North during the consumerist age, deculturation and depoliticization were becoming much more pronounced. Some, like Pier Paolo Pasolini and Guy Debord, analysed and denounced this phenomenon with varying degrees of acuity. The destruction of cities in peacetime as the new middle-class strata and immigrants were forced to move into 'peripheral' estates and social housing, and as the rise of mass marketing (supermarkets and hypermarkets), the car and television surreptitiously undermined citizenship, created a 'second people' who were almost invisible, had no voice and could be readily manipulated by the power of unscrupulous media with links to transnational companies. Globalization completed the destruction of popular culture by encouraging many people to move out of the cities and by taking away the safety nets of the welfare system. These changes encouraged the emergence of a populist political class that was corrupt, if not criminal. The 'Berlusconi phenomenon' in Italy is a caricatural example. But *berlusconization*, with or without '*Il Cavaliere*', continues to wreak havoc all over Europe, and beyond. The phenomenon of what John Kenneth Galbraith (1967) called 'satisfied majorities' occurred when the middle classes turned from solidarity to individual egoism and when Western states turned to the neo-liberal counter-revolution that dismantled the Welfare State, and it both allowed and concealed this transition. That is why the de-growth project inevitably means giving politics new foundations.

– 2 –

A Concrete Utopia

In order to live better, we now have to produce and
consume differently, to do better and more with less, by
eliminating sources of waste to begin with (for example,
unnecessary packaging, poor heat insulation, the pre-
dominance of road transport) and by increasing product
durability.

(Gorz 1994 [1991]: 106)

The De-Growth Revolution

More so than ever before, development is sacrificing populations and their concrete, local well-being on the altar of
an abstract, deterritorialized well-being. The sacrifice is
made to honour a mythical and disembodied people, and
it works, of course, to the advantage of 'the developers'
(transnational companies, politicians, technocrats and
mafias). Growth is now a profitable business only if the
costs are borne by nature, future generations, consumers'
health, wage-earners' working conditions and, above all,
the countries of the South. That is why we have
to abandon the idea of growth. Everyone, or almost

everyone, is agreed about that but no one dares to take the first step. All modern regimes have been productivist: republics, dictatorships, authoritarian systems, no matter whether their governments were of the right or the left, and no matter whether they were liberal, socialist, populist, social-liberal, social-democratic, centrist, radical or communist. They all assumed that economic growth was the unquestionable cornerstone of their systems. The change of direction that is needed is not one that can be resolved merely by an election that brings in a new government or votes in a new majority. What is needed is much more radical: a cultural revolution, nothing more and nothing less, that re-establishes politics on a new basis.

Outlining the contours of what a non-growth society might look like is an essential preliminary to any programme for political actions that respects the ecological demands of the moment.

The de-growth project is therefore a utopia, or in other words a source of hope and dreams. Far from representing a flight into fantasy, it is an attempt to explore the objective possibility of its implementation. Hence the term 'concrete utopia', in the positive sense given it by Ernst Bloch (1986 [1959]). 'Without the hypothesis that a different world is possible, there can be no politics, but only the administrative management of men and things' (Decrop 2007: 81). De-growth is therefore a political project in the strong sense of the term. It means building convivial societies that are autonomous and economical in both the North and the South. It is not, however, a political project in the electoral sense of the term. It cannot be contained within the arena of mere politicking, and is designed to restore politics to its full dignity. It is a quest for an overall theoretical coherence. Whilst it is, for the purposes of the argument, convenient to outline its stages, they should not be interpreted as stages in an agenda. The calendar comes later. The circle of the eight 'R's and their implications should be understood in that sense. We will quickly review the stages of this transformative project (and they are not the same as its concrete phases, which will be examined in chapter 3 below), and dwell at greater length on those of them that have a 'strategic' role to play. In practice – and fortunately – these stages constantly overlap and interact with one another, and that allows us to envisage a gradual process of change that may include transitions that do not figure in the theoretical schema.

The Virtuous Circle of Quiet Contraction

In the 1960s, out professors of economics and technocrats crowed over the virtuous circles of growth. That period, which was described as the *trente glorieuses*, has now given way to what critical economists are calling the *trente piteuses* [the 'piteous thirty']. Even the *trente glorieuses* were themselves what the 'planetary gardener' Gilles Clément (Clément and Jones 2006) calls the *trente disastreuses*, given the amount of damage they inflicted on both nature and humanity. The virtuous circles have ultimately proved to be somewhat perverse in more than one respect. The climate change that now threatens us is a product of our past madness. The upheavals required to build an autonomous de-growth society can, in contrast, be seen as the systematic and ambitious articulation of eight interdependent changes that reinforce one another. They can all be synthesized into a 'virtuous circles' of eight 'R's: re-evaluate, reconceptualize, restructure, redistribute, relocalize, reduce, re-use and recycle. These eight interdependent goals can trigger a process of de-growth that will be serene, convivial and sustainable.[1]

---

[1] The list of 'R's could be extended. With every, or almost every, intervention, there will be someone who proposes what he or she sees as another essential intervention such as radicalize, reconvert, redefine, reinvent (democracy), resize, remodel, rehabilitate, reduce speed, relax, render, repurchase, reimburse, renounce, re-think, and so on – but all these 'r's are, to a greater or lesser extent, implicit in the first eight.

Re-evaluate. We live in societies that are based upon the
old 'bourgeois' values of honour, public service, the transmission of knowledge, 'a good job well done', and so on.
And yet, 'It is common knowledge that these values have
become laughable . . . all that matters is the amount of
money you have pocketed, no matter how, and the number
of times you have been on television' (Castoriadis 1996:
68). To put it slightly differently, the 'underside' of the
system reveals, in Dominique Belpomme's words (2007:
220), 'an individualist megalomania, a rejection of moral-
ity, a liking for comfort, and egoism'.[2] We can immediately
see which values have to be promoted, and which values
must take precedence over the dominant values (or absence
of values) of the day. Altruism should replace egotism, and
unbridled competition should give way to cooperation.
The pleasure of leisure and the ethos of play should replace
the obsession with work. The importance of social life
should take precedence over endless consumerism, the
local over the global, autonomy over heteronomy, an
appreciation of good craftsmanship over productivist efficiency, the rational over the material, and so on. 'A concern
for truth, a sense of justice, responsibility, respect for
democracy, the celebration of differences, the duty of
solidarity and the life of the mind: these are the values
we must win back at all cost, as it is those values that
will allow us to flourish and to safeguard our future
(Belpomme 2007: 221).

The philosopher John Dewey was denouncing 'pecuni-
ary culture' and accusing the educational institution of
introducing children to the world of competition rather
than acting as a laboratory for citizenship a long time ago
(Chanial 2006). What would he have made of our com-

---

[2] He goes on: 'What do we see in the world? Lies, a two-tier legal system,
a quest for power for its own sake, a quest for money for the sake of
money, the exclusion of the poor, calumny, greed and corruption, a
caricature of democracy, the removal of the mystique surrounding
values and the worship of means that have become ends in themselves,
a denial of culture, wars, torture and, finally, the transgression of laws.'

munications society, which uses advertising to manipulate us on a vast scale? 'Just as it is difficult to see how a "consumer society" could continue to exist if it were made up of citizens whose ascetic morals led them to lead a monastic life,' writes François Brune (2006: 173), 'it is hard to imagine a de-growth society functioning with individuals whose every spontaneous and subjective impulse was still shaped by the "consumer society" 's imaginary and "way of life".'

The most important thing is to get away from the belief that we must dominate nature and to try to live in harmony with it. We have to replace the attitude of the predator with that of the gardener. For Christian ecologists, this is in fact the eleventh commandment: 'Respect nature because it is God's creation.'[3] The technological and promethean fantasy that we can create an artificial world is a way of rejecting both the world and being.[4]

Reconceptualize. A change of values allows us to see the world in a new way, and therefore to apprehend reality in a different way. We must, for instance, reconceptualize and redefine/resize the concepts of wealth and poverty; deconstructing the infernal couple of scarcity/abundance, on which the economic imaginary is based, is a matter of urgency. As Ivan Illich and Jean-Pierre Dupuy have clearly demonstrated, the economy transforms natural abundance into scarcity by creating artificial shortages and needs as it appropriates and commodifies nature (Dumouchel and Dupuy 1979; Dupuy and Robert 1976). To take the most recent illustration of this phenomenon: now that water has been privatized, living matter itself is being appropriated.

[3] On the Eleventh Commandment Fellowship developed by the theologian Paul F. Knitter, see Lanternari (2003). It is no coincidence that Knitter is also an advocate of 'religious relativism' and intercultural dialogue. For all these reasons, he has come under attack from the theocons (conservative theologians) who have had the wind in their sails since Cardinal Ratzinger was elected Pope.

[4] See Camilla Narboni's excellent doctoral thesis (2006).

GM crops are the most obvious example. Peasants are being dispossessed of the natural fertility of plants for the benefit of agri-business. 'There are no limits to the market's imagination,' remarks Bernard Maris (2006: 48). 'It nests in anything that is free, just like a cuckoo. It pushes out the other nestlings, puts its brand on everything that is free, stamps it with its logo, brands it, puts a price on it, and then sells it on.' The economists' assumptions about scarcity become a self-fulfilling prophecy, and we cannot escape the economy without facing up the challenge posed by the depletion of our natural resources.

Restructure. 'Restructuring' means adapting the productive apparatus and social relations to changing values. This restructuring will be all the more radical in that the systematic character of the dominant values will have been destabilized. What is at stake here is finding the road to a de-growth society. This raises the concrete question of getting beyond capitalism, which we will examine at the appropriate moment, and that of reconverting a productive apparatus that has to be adapted to the paradigm shift.[5]

Redistribute. Restructuring social relations automatically means redistribution. This affects how the distribution of wealth and access to the natural patrimony are distributed between North and South and, within each society, between classes, generations and individuals.

Redistribution will have a positive effect on the reduction of consumption in two ways. It will have a direct effect by reducing the power and wealth of the 'world

---

[5] Car factories, for instance, can be converted into apparatuses for recuperating energy through cogeneration. A car engine connected to an alternator and placed in a metal box is all it takes to make a micro-generator. The skills, the technologies and even the plant that are required are practically identical. Cogeneration makes it possible to increase the energy output from about 40% to 90%. It therefore reduces both the consumption of fossil energy and CO_2 emissions.

consumer class', and especially the power and wealth of the big predators. It will have an indirect effect by removing the incentives to conspicuous consumption. According to Thorstein Veblen's classic analysis (1970 [1899]),[6] the desire to consume has less to do with need than with the desire to assert our status by imitating the model of those who are just above us.

Redistributing North/South relations raises huge problems. We have contracted a huge 'ecological debt' (Attac 2006) to the South. Beginning to reduce it whilst at the same time reducing our own predation is simply a matter of fairness. As we shall see, it is not so much a matter of giving more as of taking less.[7]

Ecological footprints (which can even be broken down by types of activity and consumption) are a good way of determining each country's 'drawing rights'. 'Markets' in those rights would encourage the exchange of quotas and permits to consume. This is obviously not a way of *commodifying* nature a little more, but a way of introducing a certain suppleness into how its limitations are managed. Here, as elsewhere, the challenge is found in suiting actions to words.

Relocalize. Relocalizing means, obviously enough, producing on a local basis. Most of the products needed to meet the population's needs could be produced in local factories financed on a local basis by collective savings. All production for local needs should therefore be carried out at the local level. Whilst ideas must be able to ignore frontiers, the movement of commodities and capital must be

[6] This analysis has, fortunately, been rediscovered by Hervé Kempf (2007).

[7] What we call the rich countries' ecological debt to poor countries: the rich 'borrow' (without paying for them in the absence of heavy taxation) vast surface areas of natural resources, arable land and forest from the countries of the South. They export their pollution to the South, or at least those forms of pollution that recognize no frontiers, and not least greenhouse gases (see WWF 2006: 25).

restricted to essentials. If we wish to build a serene de-
growth society, relocalization is not just an economic
issue: politics, culture and the meaning of life must rediscover their local roots. This implies that all economic,
political and cultural decisions that can be made at the
local level must be made at that level.

Reduce. 'Reducing' means, first of all, reducing the impact
of our ways of consuming and producing on the biosphere. We must begin by reducing our habitual over-
consumption and the incredible amount we waste: 80%
of goods on the market are used only once, and then go
straight into the dustbin (Hulot 2006: 237)! The rich
countries now produce four billion tonnes of waste every
year (Maris 2006: 327). Production of domestic waste per
household is 760 kg a year in the United States, 380 kg
in France and 200 kg in most countries of the South
(Paquot 2007a: 45). Both health risks and working hours
should also be reduced. Reducing health risks implies
'precauvention' (prevention/precaution), to use Professor
Belpomme's neologism, rather than reparations – it is
worth remembering that, in 2005, French pharmacies
sold 2.6 billion boxes and phials, an increase of 8% on
the previous year.

The other thing that has to be reduced is mass tourism.
The golden age of kilometric consumerism is over. At the
moment when Richard Branson, the British billionaire
owner of Virgin, wants to put space tourism within everyone's reach (*Le Monde*, 19 April 2006), even the very
orthodox *Financial Times* admits that 'tourism will be
identified as the world's number one environmental enemy'
(Tomkins 2006).

The desire to travel and a taste for adventure are no
doubt part of human nature. They are a source of enrich-
ment that must not be allowed to dry up, but the tourist
industry has transformed legitimate curiosity and educational inquisitiveness into a consumerist consumption that
destroys the environment, culture and social fabric of the

'target' countries. 'Travelitis', or our obsession with travelling further and further, faster and faster, and more and more often (and always for less) is a largely artificial need that has been created by 'supermodern' life, exacerbated by the media and stimulated by travel agencies and tour operators, and it must be revised downwards. Whether or not 'eco-tourism', which is defined as an ethical, fair and responsible tourism and as an alternative to mass tourism, is an oxymoron that colludes with sustainable development is a legitimate question. Is it not designed to prolong the survival of a commodified, condemned and condemnable activity? The excuse that it is helping the South to develop is fallacious. According to Artisans du monde, of the 1,000 euros spent on a holiday package, less than 200 euros remains in the host country. The coming oil shortage and climate change promise us a very different future: not so far, less often, slower and ever more expensive. Truth to tell, this is becoming tragic only because of the emptiness and disenchantment that mean that, whilst we live to an increasing extent in virtual reality, we travel in real time, and at the planet's expense. We have to relearn the wisdom of past ages: enjoy slowness and appreciate our own territory.

> Going travelling was once an adventure that was full of the unexpected in terms of the time it might take and all the uncertainties, and not least the uncertainty of coming home. . . . But most people had no incentive to travel and stayed where they were. A steeple in the centre and a horizon that marked the boundaries of a territory were enough for a lifetime. We can choose between thousands of possibilities, but choosing to stay in the place where we happen to have been born does not necessarily mean that we have no imagination. It can even mean the very opposite. You do not have to travel to allow the imagination to take wing. (Revel 2005: 119)

Unlike the 705 Papuan peoples, who have been doomed for thousands of years to live the whole of human experience within the limited horizons of their canton, we, thanks to the wonders of technology, have the unprecedented good fortune to be able to travel in virtual reality without leaving home. And after all, adventurous souls can always windsurf to the Seychelles . . . if the islands have not been swallowed up by the sea.

Shortening the working week is, finally, an essential element, as we shall see when we discuss policies for fighting unemployment. This obviously means job-sharing to ensure that anyone who wants a job can find one. A shorter working week must go hand in hand with the possibility of changing one's job as the economic situation changes or at different times in one's personal life. According to Willem Hoogendijk (2003), types of activity should be diversified: 'If demand for shoes or TVs drops off . . . then production at the respective plants will simply be cut back for a while, freeing up the staff and workers for other activities.'[8] Wage-earners could work in agriculture or commercial garden centres or on building sites. They could work in the transport sector, in education or on sports schemes for disturbed adolescents. As is obvious from what they do with their spare time, most people have talents that extend far beyond the jobs they usually do for a living. Although the unions are, for the moment and for understandable reasons, hostile to them, temp agencies, which are popular with both employers and workers – because of the variety of jobs they offer – represent a step in the right direction. We just have to see them in a different light.

Above all, we must be weaned off our addiction to 'the job', as it is a major element in the tragedy of productivism. We will not be able to build a serene de-growth society unless we rediscover the repressed dimensions of life: the leisure to do one's duty as a citizen, the pleasure of the freedom to engage in freely chosen arts and crafts

[8] I am grateful to Willem Hogendijk for supplying me with a copy of his paper (Translator).

activities, the sensation of having found time to play, contemplate, meditate, enjoy conversations or quite simply to enjoy being alive.[9]

Re-use/recycle. No one in their right mind would deny that we have to reduce conspicuous waste, fight the built-in obsolescence of appliances, and recycle waste that cannot be re-used directly. The possibilities are endless, and many have been tested on a small scale. The Swiss firms Rohner and Design Tex have, for example, developed and produced an upholstery fabric that is naturally degradable once it has reached the end of its life cycle. Other companies have developed carpets made of organic materials that can be used as mulch for parks when they are worn out. The German chemicals giant BASF has developed a fabric made from nylon fibre that can be recycled indefinitely and that breaks down – when the product to which it gave birth had worn out – into its basic elements, which can then be re-used in new products. In 1990, Xerox – a company specializing in photocopiers – developed a programme that allows products to be seen as an assemblage of parts that can be recycled when they have reached the end of their useful life. When its copiers are returned to it, Xerox undertakes to re-use most of the raw materials from which they are made (Bevilacqua 2006: 129). Once again, what is missing is the incentive that will put both manufacturers and consumers on the 'virtuous' path. And yet it is easy to come up with such incentives; we simply lack the political will to implement them.

[9]'*Liberated time* [*le temps libéré*] is not "*free time*" [*temps libre*] – which is immediately captured by the leisure and health industries – but a reconciliation with oneself, and it can sometimes be tense and contradictory,' writes Thierry Paquot (2007: 65). 'Liberated time is by no means a left-over – what is "left" after the time that is spent travelling to work, work itself, and the time we devote to shopping, to our families and so on. It is a demand, like the demand for human dignity, for the least incomplete possible control over one's own destiny.'

All this points the way towards a utopia in the best sense of the term. This utopia is an intellectual construct that functions on an ideal basis, but it is also concrete in the sense that it takes as its starting point elements that already exist and changes that can be implemented. If we want it, we can have another world that is at once desirable, necessary and possible.

Within this project, autonomy has to be understood in the strong and etymological sense of the term (*autonomos*: 'He who establishes his own norms') and as a reaction against the heteronomy of the 'invisible hand' of the market, the dictatorship of financial markets and the diktats technoscience issue to (super-)modern society. This autonomy does not imply boundless freedom. As Aristotle reminds us, we have to learn to obey before we can learn how to command. In a society of free citizens, 'learning' to obey has to be understood as meaning serving an apprenticeship, as a non-servile obedience to the law we have chosen to obey (servile obedience is an apprenticeship in tyranny). There is no denying that voluntary servitude can be enjoyable in both cases. When it comes to 'consumption', the dividing line between an instrumental usage that respects individuals and an instrumentalization that does not is both tenuous and problematic. The existence of efficient forms of reciprocity marks all the difference between the two forms. This is one of the many challenges that a democratic society always has to face. Hence the importance of conviviality.

Conviviality, which Ivan Illich (1972) borrows from the great eighteenth-century French gourmet Brillat-Savarin,[10] is designed to reknit the social bond that has been unravelled by what Arthur Rimbaud called the 'horrors of economics'. Conviviality reintroduces the spirit of the gift into trade, alongside the law of the jungle, and thus restores the link with Aristotle's *philia* ('friendship').

---

[10] Jean-Anthelme Brillat-Savarin (1755–1825): author of *La Physiologie du gout ou Méditations de gastronomie transcendante* (English edn: 1970 [1825]).

Some will no doubt see the systematic recourse to the prefix 're' in the eight 'R's as the hallmark of a reactionary way of thinking, or as a romantic or nostalgic desire to go back to living in the past. Let me simply say that, leaving aside a certain flirtatiousness on the author's part (placing its stages under the sign of the letter 'R'), the actions in question are as much part of a revolution as a backward move, and are at once innovative and repetitive. If there is an element of reaction, it is a reaction to the system's excesses and hubris – which finds expression in the many 'overs' that Jean-Paul Besset denounces, and which should be replaced by 're's, over-development, over-production, over-abundance, over-extraction, over-fishing, over-grazing, over-consumption, over-packaging, over-communications, too much traffic [*surcirculation*], over-medicalization, over-indebtedness, over-supply . . . (Besset 2005: 182).[11] As Michael Singleton remarks (2006: 53), this over-speeding thermo-industrial system is doing more and more damage, which we can sum up in 'a growing list of words beginning with the prefix "de": industrial delocalization, monetary deflation, political disenchantment [*désenchantement*], cultural demotivation and religious demystification. Whatever else we do,' he adds, 'we have to ensure that the "de" in de-growth echoes the "putting off the inevitable" to which the original Latin *dis* lends itself so well.' At the centre of the virtuous circles of the eight 'R's cultural revolution, there is another 'R' that is implicit in all of them: resist.

De-Growth as a Local Project

It might be said that all eight 'R's are equally important. It seems to me, however, that three of them have a 'strategic' role: re-evaluation, because it determines all changes, reduction, because it is a condensation of all the practical

[11] Besset then adds: 'Overdoses harm living things. Overdoing things destroys individuals.'

imperatives of de-growth, and relocalization, because it concerns the everyday lives and jobs of millions of people.[12] Relocalization therefore has a central role to play in our concrete utopia, and almost immediately suggests a political programme. De-growth appears to give a new life to the ecologists' old slogan of 'Think globally, act locally'. Whilst the utopia of de-growth implies thinking at a global level, its realization begins at grassroots level. There are two interdependent sides to the local de-growth project: political innovation and economic autonomy.

Inventing Local Ecological Democracy

One solution to the urban and political peripheralization generated by the growth society might be a return to Murray Bookchin's 'utopia' of 'ecomunicipalism' (Bookchin 1980). Bookchin envisaged here an ecological society made up of a municipality of municipalities, each in turn made up of a commune of small communes, in perfect harmony with their ecosystems (Magnaghi 2006: 100). The reconquest or reinvention of 'commons' (common goods, common spaces) and self-organized 'bioregions' might be one illustration of this approach (Esteva 2004; Esteva and Prakash 1998). A bioregion or ecoregion, defined as a coherent spatial entity that expresses a geographical, social and historical reality, might be predominantly rural or predominantly urban. An urban bioregion could be described as a municipality of municipalities, a 'town of towns' or even a 'town of villages', or in other words an ecopolis, meaning a polycentric or multipolar network (Magnaghi 2006: 69–112). A bioregion consists of a complex set of local territorial systems with a high capacity for an ecological self-sustainability designed to

[12] 'Four themes can structure the future space of sober societies: local and regional self-sufficiency, the geographical decentralization of powers, economic relocalization and protectionism, concerted planning and rationing,' remarks Yves Cochet (2005: 208).

reduce external diseconomies and energy consumption (Bonora 2006).

According to some, this puts us in a 'democratic dilemma' that might be summed up thus: the smaller the political entity/unit and the more direct control its citizens have, the more restricted its domains of sovereignty (Dahl 1983). Its capacity for decision-making and action cannot apply to questions that extend beyond its territorial limits, and will be influenced by external dynamics (Bonora 2006: 113), especially in the ecological domain. As its territorial political constituency expands, on the other hand, its citizens will have fewer opportunities to participate in decision-making. That is a truism, but Paola Bonora suggests that we should approach the question in terms of identity rather than size. What matters is the existence of a collective project rooted in a territory, defined as a place for communal living that must be protected and cared for the good of all. Participation, which is then implicit in action, becomes the 'guardian and promoter of the spirit of the place' (Bonora 2006: 114). Size is no longer a topographical problem, but a social problem. We are talking about a space with a recognizable identity and a capacity for coordinated collective action. Bookchin's idea that a metropolitan area could be an articulated set of autonomous neighbourhoods that function as juxtaposed communes is interesting, but it can work only if the neighbourhood councils have real power and are not just transmission belts.

The 'new communes' network in Italy is certainly one of the most original and most promising initiatives.[13] This is an association made up of researchers, social movements and many local politicians from small communes, but also from larger entities such as the province of Milan and the Tuscany region which are trying to solve the problems generated by the excesses of the growth society at the local

[13] The 'commune' is the smallest administrative unit in the Italian and French systems of local government (Translator).

level and in honest ways. The most original feature of the network, whose meeting in Bari in October 2005 was attended by five hundred participants, lies in its choice of a strategy based upon a territory. The 'local', in other words, is seen as a field where social actors, a physical environment and territorial patrimonies can interact. According to the network's charter, this is 'a political project that values local resources and specificities, encourages processes of conscious and responsible autonomy, and refuses to be steered from outside by the invisible hand of the global market (hetero-leadership)'.[14] It is, in other words, a laboratory for a critical analysis, and for self-government and the defence of common goods. The experiment has a lot in common with the 'urban village' idea and with the example set by the 'slow city' movements.[15] This movement complements the slow food movement, which has been joined by 100,000 producers, peasants, artisans and fishermen all over the world in order to fight the standardization of food and to rediscover taste and local specialities (Petrini 2006). Although it has put down deep roots, this local project is neither closed nor egotistical; 'on the contrary, it presupposes openness and a generous idea of giving and taking' (Bonora 2006: 118).

The de-growth society implies a high level of protectionism against unbridled and unfair competition, but it also implies a great openness towards 'spaces' that adopt comparable measures. If, as Michel Torga was already saying in 1954, 'the universal is the local without walls', we can deduce that the local, conversely, is the universal plus frontiers, boundaries, buffer zones, smugglers, interpreters and translators. An identity that has been chosen, that is

[14] Carta del Nouvo Municipio; see *www.nouvomuncipo.org* and *www. communivirtuosi.org.*
[15] This is a global network of medium-sized towns established in the wake of the slow food movement. They deliberately restrict their demographic growth to 60,000 inhabitants. Beyond that limit, it would be impossible to use the terms 'local' and 'slow'.

to a greater or lesser extent plural and that is still bound up with a shared vision of its destiny, is an essential element in guaranteeing a bioregional unit its consistency.[16] Michael Singleton notes that there is a great danger that anyone who uses the words 'local' and 'community', and who casts doubt on the possibility or opportuneness of an abstract political universalism (which is code for world government),

> will be called all the names that Modernity has anathemized: fascism, nationalism, male chauvinism, paternalism, elitism, nostalgia for the past. . . . How can we get people to understand that de-growth is not a return to the fetters of comunitarianism (the small nuclear family, the posh area, regional egotism . . .), but to an organic 're-weaving' of the local (allowing people to spend more time together, as they did until the 1960s, thanks to, amongst other things, village schools, 'family' firms, local shops and local cinemas rather than spending their days shuttling between schools, industrial zones and out-of-town supermarkets)? (Singleton 2006: 52)

From this point of view, the local is not a closed microcosm, but a knot in a network of virtuous and interdependent transversal relations, with a view to experimenter practices that can strengthen democracy (including participatory budgets) and make it possible to resist the dominance of neo-liberalism.

Rediscovering Local Economic Autonomy

The relocalization project implies a quest for self-sufficiency in food and then economic and financial self-sufficiency. Every region's basic activity should be protected

---

[16] Whilst language is, as Martin Heidegger said, the 'dwelling place of beings', 'Babelization', according to Thierry Paquot (2006: 181), 'guarantees not only cultural diversity but also a diversity of ways of being and ways of thinking.'

and developed, including forms of agriculture and horticulture, preferably organic, that respect the passage of the seasons.[17] Willem Hoogendijk (2003) looks at the interesting example of Holland:

> According to calculations by the Dutch Agricultural Economic Institute (LEI) back in 1980, agricultural self-sufficiency was then a viable option for the Netherlands, one of the most densely populated countries in the world. More recently the LEI calculated – to the great surprise of even the researchers – that all 16 million of us could now eat domestically grown *organic* food (while reducing our meat consumption and eating more seasonable produce).

He then goes on to describe what this new model for agriculture would look like:

> Extensive, outdoor agriculture on mixed farms (with livestock and arable farming combined where possible or at least adjacent, so the manure can be spread back on the farm or on the neighbour's). Extensive horticulture, too, with all the conserving and drying of produce and other work it entails. Then there's our waste, including in the long run our faeces, to return to the land as fertilizer, fodder or soil conditioner. By taking out 'food subscriptions' with individual farmers and helping out with the harvest (as is already done throughout the world) we can forge closer bonds between farmers/growers and consumers of their produce. And that food will be fresh and healthy, too, subject to lower costs and taxes because of less storage and refrigeration and transport.

Such autonomy does not necessarily mean complete autarky: 'There can be trade with regions that have likewise "dropped out" : balanced trade that respected regional

[17] 'Striving for the most complete possible national and then regional self-sufficiency, by guaranteeing peasants and adequate income and encouraging the revival of rural communities based upon peasant, sustainable and organic agriculture' (Cochet 2005: 224).

independence: i.e. mutual trading of regional surpluses without overstretching people or systems (TVs for dates, butter for olives and so on).'

We can also achieve local autonomy in terms of energy: renewable energies 'are well adapted to decentralized societies in which there are no large concentrations of human beings. But population dispersal is also an advantage: every region in the world has a natural potential to develop one or more form of renewable energy' (Cochet 2005: 140).

Local shops will be encouraged: the creation of one precarious job in the mass market destroys five sustainable jobs in local shops (Jacquiau 2006). According to the French National Institute for Statistics and Economic Studies (INSEE), the appearance of supermarkets (at the end of the 1960s) did away with 17% of bakers in France (17,800), 84% of grocers (73,800) and 43% of hardware dealers (4,300). A significant proportion of local life was destroyed, and much of the social fabric was undone (Ridoux 2006: 11). Given that the big supermarkets' five central purchasing departments now account for 90% of France's retail trade, we've got a lot on our plate.

We must also come up with a real local monetary policy.

If the inhabitants' purchasing power is to be maintained, monetary flows must, as far as possible, remain within the region, whilst economic decisions must be taken at the regional level, as far as possible. We have an expert's word for it (the expert in question is one of the inventors of the euro, as it happens): 'Encouraging local or regional development whilst keeping a monopoly on the national currency is like trying to dry out an alcoholic by giving him gin.' (Bernard Lietaer, cited Blanc 2006: 76)

The role of local, social or complementary currencies has to be related to unsatisfied needs with regard to resources which would otherwise go unused. There have been countless micro-experiments ranging from the cheques used in local exchange systems, 'free money', Argentina's *creditos*, to vouchers for specific purposes (transport, meals and *fuereai kippu* in Japan – 'fraternal relations coupons' for health care for the elderly). And yet no systematic attempt has ever been made to reappropriate the creation and use of local currencies. The bioregion would probably be the ideal scale for such experiments. And no doubt we will have to think about inventing 'bioregional currencies'.

To sum up, regionalization means: less transport, transparent production lines, incentivizing sustainable production and consumption, reducing dependency upon capital flow and multinationals, and greater security in every sense of the word. Regionalizing the economy and embedding it in local societies protects the environment, and the environment is, in the last analysis, the basis for any economy. Regionalization facilitates a more democratic approach to the economy, reduces unemployment, increases participation (and therefore integration), encourages solidarity, opens up new perspectives for the developing countries and, finally, improves the health of citizens in the rich countries by encouraging sobriety and reducing stress (Hoogendijk 2003).

Local De-Growth Initiatives

The necessary changes in world 'governance' have yet to come about, and governments that have been won over to the de-growth cause have yet to be elected, but many local actors have, either implicitly or explicitly, set off down the road to the fertile utopia of de-growth. Local collectives from North Carolina to Chalon-sur-Saône are showing the way and are implementing plans to fight climate change. The example of Bed ZED (Beddington Zero Energy Development) has established a model for reducing energy consumption. Some regions (Upper Austria, Tuscany and even Poland) have decided to reject GM crops. Orders from local authorities and state-owned establishments (schools, hospitals, etc.) account for a significant proportion of public spending (12% of GDP in France), and can therefore be used to popularize the idea of converting the whole economy to ecology. Adapting their terms and conditions would be enough to encourage their beneficiaries to adopt good environmental practices (Canfin 2006: 72). Local authorities can ensure that the establishments under their control rely primarily on local firms and suppliers (Chambéry), insist that public canteens and restaurants use biological agricultural produce (Lorinet, Pamiers), use mechanical or thermal weeding techniques, and not pesticides, to maintain public spaces (roadside verges and green spaces), as they have done in Rennes, Grenoble and Mulhouse, and use compost instead of chemical fertilizers (Hulot 2006: 170). Several regions in France are encouraging the use of public transport: the Rhône-Alpes regional council, for example, points out that since 1997, 400 extra trains have been introduced, 115 stations have been renovated and that 60% of the infrastructure has been updated. Passenger numbers have risen from between 5 to 6% as a result (Ridoux 2006: 86).

> We must immediately become involved in municipal life by taking part in elections, attending council meetings, and becoming members of citizens' associations that encourage other aspects of sobriety: more room for pedestrians and cyclists and less for cars; a greater variety of local shops and fewer supermarkets; more small blocks of flats and fewer towers; more local services, less urban zoning, etc. (Cochet 2005: 200)

Whilst there are obvious limitations to local projects, we should not under-estimate the potential for political advances at the local level. The experience of the commune of Mouans-Sartoux is interesting: thanks to the efforts of its mayor, André Aschieri, the station was reopened and a new train service was introduced, more 'public utilities' have been brought under local authority control (water, transport and even funeral parlours), cycle routes and green spaces have been developed, support has been given to local farmers and small shopkeepers. The commune has rejected the advances of property speculators and supermarkets, and has avoided the 'suburbanization' that would have been seen as inevitable thirty years ago. The annual literary festival is a vibrant symbol of its new vivacity.

As Yves Cochet has suggested (2005: 224), the WTO should be replaced by a WLO (World Localization Organization), and its slogan should be 'Global protection for the local'.

Is Reducing Growth a Retrograde Step?

When it is possible, beating a retreat is, in some domains, a sign of wisdom. Especially when it comes to food supplies. In the OECD countries, the current trend is for food that it less local, less seasonal, less reliant on vegetables, and less expensive. And yet in recent years, the regions of France have become more food-dependent. Take the example of Limousin, which is regarded as a rural region. According to Emmanuel Bailly (2006), only 10% of all food is produced and processed locally. 'Almost no potatoes are now grown, and the surface area devoted to the crop has fallen from 7,400 hectares to about 300 hectares. . . . In 1970, almost 6,300 hectares were devoted to growing vegetables; the figure for 2000 was 300 hectares (6,700 tonnes). Regional production meets only 8.1% of the population's demand for fresh vegetables.' Limousin's golden delicious apples now have to face competition from Chinese apples that are twice as cheap, shipping costs included! And before long, local beef will have to face competition from beef on the hoof from South America. That is already happening with packaged meat. Production has been delocalized by the shareholders in the big chains, which are supplied by purchasing departments that buy from outside the region. These practices are making the system very fragile. When the seamen's strike called by the Société Nationale Maritime Corse Méditerranée block-aded Corsica in October 2005, the island began to run out of supplies of vegetables and fresh produce after four to five days. Whilst they border on the caricatural, the travels of Danish prawns are not, unfortunately, exceptional. They go to Morocco to be peeled and then back to Denmark before being sent to market. What is, if possible, still more aberrational is that Scottish langoustines are expatriated to Thailand to be peeled by hand in a Findus factory and then returned to Scotland to be cooked before being sold in Marks and Spencer's stores. Reversing this trend would reduce wastage and would make our supply chains, and especially the food chain, less vulnerable to the rising cost of energy and the growing shortage of hydrocarbons (Cochet 2005: 97). According to Yves Cochet (2005: 89), the outcome would be 'food supplies that use less energy and reverse three current trends: supplies would be more local, more seasonal and more dependent upon vegeta-bles'. They will remain 'more expensive' if we go on making the victims pay and subsidizing the polluters.

Once again, a certain decolonization of the imaginary is required. Whilst they do not necessarily worship prog-ress and modernity (which we all do to some extent), 'decent people' are obsessed with a fear of going back-wards, which would mean poverty and humiliation for them. 'When I was a boy,' a Sicilian friend told me, 'I was the only one of my friends to have shoes. Everyone else played football barefoot. Nowadays, all the children have shoes. And we have growth to thank for that.' 'Objectors to growth' often clash with 'objectors to de-growth' who make similar comments, and there is no denying their validity. Their fear of being plunged back into a wretched past is, no matter how distorted their memories may be, quite legitimate. But no one is suggesting that we have to go back to that destitution, which was usually exacerbated by intolerable inequalities. We do, however, have to ask ourselves if the experience of well-being necessarily requires us to have ten pairs of shoes, which are often of poor quality, rather than two pairs that will last. Murray Bookchin (2001) rejects the suggestion that the good life requires us to have limitless personal material goods, and counters libertarians' imagined opposition to this infringement of 'autonomy' by asserting that acceptable needs should be determined by the community as a whole.

Willem Hoogendijk (2003) tries to argue the case for the self-limitation of needs. According to the economics textbooks, there are no limits to our so-called 'needs', but Hoogendijk argues that a clearer distinction should be made between what Keynes called primary and secondary needs. There are naturally limits to the former, but not to the latter. Hoogendijk suggests that we make a distinction between basic or normal needs and other needs. The former (food, clothing, housing, work and sociability/sex) can become unreasonable (more space per person, more pairs of shoes, more central heating, etc.) but they are, in relative terms, subject to saturation. The latter are promoted by the growth society, which relies upon the dynamics of the endless creation of needs, and can be classified as:

- the need to compensate for past losses, such as the loss of green spaces to the cars that invade our streets, of quiet places and of swimming pools to replace polluted rivers, and so on;
- the need to repair or prevent damage, to purify our air and water and to lime forests affecting by acid rain; this leads to the emergence of an expanding eco-industry;
- other needs created by earlier developments: new jobs are needed to replace those that have been lost to automation; we need more transport because the physical organization of space is based upon separation; unbridled competition means that we need machines that can produce goods more quickly.

One of the objectives of the system is to create needs and then to satisfy them by producing goods to mend what has been broken and to compensate and console us for what we have lost. Reducing growth also means slowing down, and therefore resisting both the empire of speed and current trends. The recent abolition of the siesta in Spain is symptomatic of the absurdity of the growth society. 'The arbitrary abolition of the siesta in order to bring Spain into line with the working hours of branches of transnational firms (I am thinking here of the Spanish banking system which has adopted European opening hours) is,' remarks Thierry Paquot (2006: 178), 'an act of considerable symbolic violence, and also a counter-productive measure.' And all doctors are indeed agreed that this ancestral practice has beneficial effects.

All in all, it is not a question of making consumers feel guilty in order to convert them to asceticism, but of making them more responsible citizens.

The recipe for de-growth lies in doing more, and doing better, with less. Illich's formula must not be understood in the sense of economic rationalization, as the technocratic caricature would have us believe. The dismantling of the Welfare State and the budget cuts that followed has led to the emergence of new forms of management in the public sector, and they are replacing the rationalization of budgetary choices. The goal is now to improve the results of social policy by spending less by using associations (or even the voluntary sector) that can compete in the market for subsidies. The spirit of de-growth is as far removed as it could be from the obsessional search to make savings of all kinds and from the underlying neo-liberal ideology and its key words (efficiency, performance, excellence, short-term profitability, cost-cutting, flexibility, return on investments, etc.). That leads to destruction of the social fabric. Of course the goal is to consume less of the planet's limited natural resources, but to use them so as to produce an

extra-economic surplus; de-growth is therefore the dia-
metrical opposite of the goal of the technocrats.

Does this imply rationing? Some are seriously thinking
of rationing where energy and the emission of greenhouse
gases are concerned, even if rationing is reminiscent of a
wartime economy. But it might well be said that we are
involved in a battle for humanity's survival. Lester Brown
(2004) notes that in 1942, and faced with a wartime emergency, the American economy could convert car plants to
produce tanks overnight. Reconverting the same car industry to produce microgenerators might represent a similar
challenge. In emergency conditions, a democratic country
like the United Kingdom was prepared to accept a programme of blood, sweat and tears. Far from necessarily
implying such sacrifices, the ecological conversion of our
societies holds out the promise of more *joie de vivre*, and
for today rather than tomorrow: healthier food, more
leisure time and more conviviality.

Given that we can reasonably count on an increase in
ecological efficiency (greater biocapacity, more productive
farmland, fisheries and forests) thanks to better technologies and better management, there will be less need to
reduce.[18] We can, in other words, get back to the 'right'
ecological footprint (one planet), which means cutting the
depletion of natural resources by 30%, by reducing 'final'
consumption by 50%. The improvement in our quality of
life would be out of all proportion to the measures that
are needed.

De-Growth: A Challenge for the South

Paradoxically, the idea of de-growth was, in a sense, born
in the South and, more specifically, in Africa. The project
for an autonomous and economical society in fact emerged
from the critique of development.

[18] By about 30% by 2100, according to the WWF.

For over forty years, a small anti- or post-developmentalist 'internationale' has been analysing and denouncing the harmful effect of development in Africa, from Boumédienne's Algeria to Nyerere's Kenya (see Sachs 1992). Its critique applies not only to capitalist or ultra-liberal development, as in Ivory Coast, but also to what is officially known as 'socialist', participatory', 'endogenous', self-reliant or 'popular' development, which has often been implemented or supported by humanist NGOs. Although there have been a few remarkable micro-successes, development has been a massive failure and what was meant to improve the quality of everyone's life has resulted in corruption, incoherence and structural adjustment plans that have turned poverty into misery.

A critique addressed to the South supplies the *historic* alternative, namely self-organized societies and vernacular economies (see Latouche 1998). These analyses naturally take an interest in alternative initiatives in the North such as LES (local exchange systems), REPAS (*réseaux d'échange des pratiques alternatives et solidaires*), *Banche del tempo* (individual exchange of services), cooperatives, and so on, but not in a societal alternative in the singular. The fact that the environmental crisis has coincided with the emergence of globalization, together with the unexpected – but very relative – success of the critics of development, who seemed for a long time to be preaching in the wilderness, means that we have to look more closely at what this critique implies for the economy and society of the North. The farce of sustainable development in fact concerns both the North and the South, and growth now poses a global threat. Hence the de-growth proposal.

Reducing Africa's ecological footprint (and GDP) is neither necessary nor desirable. But we should not therefore conclude that a growth society should be built there. De-growth concerns the countries of the South to the extent that they have committed themselves to building growth economies and that de-growth can prevent them from being trapped in the blind alley into which that adventure is leading them. Far from unreservedly singing the praises of the informal economy, I think that the societies of the South can, if there is still time, 'undevelop' themselves, or in other words avoid the obstacles that prevent them from realizing their full potential. First of all, it is clear that de-growth in the North is a precondition for the success of any form of alternative in the South. So long as Ethiopia and Somalia are forced to export foodstuffs to feed our animals when famine is raging, and so long as we go on fattening our livestock on soja cattlecake that is produced by burning the Amazonian forest, we will asphyxiate any attempt at real autonomy in the South.[19]

If we dare to implement de-growth in the South, we can attempt to trigger a spiral moment that will bring us into the orbit of the virtuous circles of the three 'R's. The spiral that leads to de-growth could be organized around alternative and complementary 'R's, such as *Rompre* [break], Renew, Rediscover, Reintroduce, Recuperate, and so on. Break away from economic and cultural dependency on the North. Renew contact with the thread of a history that was interrupted by colonization, development and globalization. Rediscover and reappropriate the cultural identity of the South. Reintroduce specific products that have been forgotten or abandoned, and 'anti-economic' values that are bound up with the past of these countries. Recuperate traditional technologies and skills.

In February 2007, the Italian NGO Chiama l'Africa organized a debate on the theme of 'poverty and de-growth' with some intellectuals from Benin at the Emmaüs Centre in Tohue, near Cotonou, with Albert Tévoédjrè as the keynote speaker. The debate summed up the 'African paradox'.

---

[19] Not to mention the fact that global 'relocation' helped to accelerate climate change a little more, or that speculative *latifundista* agriculture in Brazil is depriving the poor of beans, and that there is also the danger of biogenetic disasters such as 'mad cow' disease.

No one remembers Albert Tévoédjrè. And yet, at the suggestion of Ivan Illich, he published a best-selling book that anticipated the idea of de-growth in 1978. His *Poverty: Wealth of Mankind* (Tévoédjrè 1979) criticizes the absurdity of cultural and industrial mimetism, celebrates sobriety, which is part of the African tradition, denounces the excesses of the consumer society, with its deliberate creation of artificial needs, the dehumanization generated by the dominance of cash-based relations, and its destruction of the environment. He advocates, finally, a return to self-sufficiency at the village level.

Now in his late eighties and still in good health, the man has not reneged on his ideas, but they are no longer of any interest to anyone in Africa. Like many African intellectuals he has, perhaps in vain, devoted his energies to politics, but has never been able to act on his convictions while holding ministerial office.

In *L'Autre afrique* (Latouche 1998), I analyse how those who are excluded from economic modernity can organize themselves by 'making do'. They provide an example of how a society that is autonomous, economical and sustainable can be built in conditions that are much more precarious than any that might be experienced by de-growth societies in the North without owing anything, or while owing almost nothing, to the continent's intellectual and political elites. This ability not only to survive but also to construct a complete life in the margins of the global market society is based upon three kinds of *bricolage*: an imaginary *bricolage* with the proliferation of syncretic cults and sects (even in Muslim countries, with their brotherhoods and dissident groups); techno-economic *bricolage*, thanks to an ingenious, industrious and entrepreneurial recuperation (as opposed to Western economic rationality, which is based upon engineering, industrial and entrepreneurial rationality); and above all social *bricolage*, thanks to the invention of neo-clan bonds (resulting from simultaneous membership of a host of associations).

Although this is a real alternative society that has yet to gain recognition or appear on the political and international stage, it is, however, under constant threat from a triumphant and arrogant globalization (even when it is in crisis). Whilst we have witnessed its surprising 'success', the colonization of the imaginary, which has already corrupted 'official Africa', now poses a threat to the other Africa. The invasion of the international media thanks to radio, television, the Internet and mobile phones is having a corrosive effect on the social bond. One has only to think of the young people who want to leave their own countries, which they have come to see as hell, for the artificial paradises of the North, even though they will find that the door is locked against them. The salvage dealers who triumphed over European manufactured exports now sometimes have to compete with very cheap mass-produced Chinese consumer goods. Whilst those goods are not generating a true individualism, the processes of individuation are successfully undermining the solidarity on which the alternative world was based. Pollution, finally, is no respecter of frontiers and is making a degraded environment more and more unliveable. Like a cancer, a veritable second-hand consumer society, with battered old cars, broken mobile phones and computers undergoing repairs and everything else the West has thrown away, is eating away at Africa's ability to resist. It is to be hoped that the crisis hits the North in time to give the other Africa a chance. A few years ago, old ladies in Benin's villages would say to me: 'When are you French coming back? We've suffered too much since you left.' Nowadays, young people bombard us with other questions: 'Help us get to France. There's no hope for us here.' Tragically, the African paradox is very similar to the Western paradox. As my late friend Jean Baudrillard once wrote (2005): 'The only thing that keeps Western culture going is the fact that the rest of the world wants to be part of it.'

If we really want the North's concern for justice to extend beyond the need to reduce its 'ecological footprint', we should perhaps extend its ecological debt to include another 'debt'. Native peoples sometimes remind us that the North has a debt of restitution. Repaying the debt of the South's lost honour (the loss of its plundered heritage is much more problematic) might mean entering into a de-growth partnership with the South.

Conversely, persevering with or, worse still, introducing the logic of growth into the South on the grounds that it will lift these wretched countries out of the poverty that has been created by growth itself cannot but Westernize them still further. The suggestion that we should 'build schools, health centres, systems that provide water that is fit to drink, and get back to self-sufficiency in food' (Harribey 2004) reflects good intentions on the part of our friends in the anti-globalization movement, but it also reflects the usual ethnocentrism of development. We have two options. We can ask the countries concerned what they want by consulting their governments or organizing opinion polls that will be manipulated by the media. It is obvious what answer we will get. Rather than meeting the 'basic needs' Western paternalism ascribes to them, they will ask for air-conditioning units, mobile phones, refrigerators and especially cars, along with nuclear power stations, Rafale jets and AMX tanks to keep the politicians happy. . . Or we can listen to this cry from the heart from a Guatemalan peasant leader: 'Leave the poor alone and stop talking to them about development' (Gras 2003: 249). All leaders of popular movements, from Vandana Shiva in India to Emmanuel Ndione in Senegal, say the same thing in different ways. Ultimately, the reason why 'getting back to self-sufficiency in food' is undeniably a matter of urgency in the countries of the South is that they have lost their self-sufficiency. Africa was still self-sufficient until the 1960s, which is when the great development offensive began. Surely it is the imperialism of colonization, development and globalization that destroyed the self-sufficiency of the countries of the South and that is exacerbating their dependency day by day? Before it was so grossly polluted by industrial waste, their water was usually drinkable, with or without taps. As for schools and health centres, can such institutions really promote and defend culture and health? Ivan Illich (1971, 1977) had serious doubts about their relevance to the North. Where the South is concerned, even greater circumspection is required, as some (though no doubt too few . . .) intellectuals from those countries are saying. The solicitude of the White Man who worries about de-growth with the noble aim of coming to their aid is suspect. As Majid Rahnema rightly points out (2003: 268),

> What we go on calling *aid* is no more than spending that is designed to reinforce the structures that generate poverty. On the other hand, the victims who have been robbed of their wealth never receive any aid when they try to distance themselves from the globalized productive system and try to find alternatives that are in keeping with their own aspirations.

And yet the alternative to development, in both the South and the North, cannot be either an impossible return to the past or a uniform de-growth model that is imposed from on high. For the excluded and those who have been ship-wrecked by development, it has to be a sort of synthesis of traditions that have been lost and a modernity to which they have been denied access. That paradoxical formula is a good summary of the twofold challenge they face. Once their creativity and ingenuity have been freed from the shackles of economism and 'developmentalism', the odds are that their remarkable social inventiveness will be able to meet it. Post-development, which has to be plural, means looking for forms of collective prosperity that do not put the emphasis on a material well-being that destroys the environment and the social bond. The objective of 'the good life' can take many different forms, depending on the context. The point is, in other words, that we have to reconstruct/rediscover new cultures.

Once again, we are talking about a concrete, fertile utopia, and not a political agenda. Chapter 3 will not present an agenda for building autonomous societies in the South because I take the view that the content of the project must be determined by the populations concerned. Attempting to implement it in the South will certainly come up against many obstacles. 'If you think of a lion, climb a tree,' says the Bantu proverb. Whilst anyone who embarks upon such a political project in the North risks assassination, even thinking about it in the South means that they will suffer the same fate as Patrice Lumumba, Thomas Sankara or Salvador Allende. According to Pierre Gevaert (2005: 97–8), who has thought a lot about this issue,

> Africans, in particular, have yet to become slaves to modern comfort, and should bear in mind the following points:
> 1. Do not rely too much on the false wealth of the West, and try to be as autonomous of it as possible.
> 2. Replace some foreign paper currencies (CFA francs, dollars, pounds stirling) with a local exchange currency inspired by the LES.
> 3. Put a gradual end to monoculture for export and replace it with food crops that are not dependent on inputs from abroad (chemical fertilizers, pesticides, etc.) by using compost that uses every wisp of corn, dung and other organic materials.
> 4. When harvests produce a surplus, try to transform the raw materials themselves so as to avoid involvement in unequal markets, and take advantage of the value added generated by their transformations (e.g. sesame or groundnut paste).
> 5. Protect your land and soil by surrounding plots with anti-erosion 'mini-ditches'.
> 6. Use the sun for cooking. Use solar ovens; a local carpenter can make them for 100 euros at most.
> 7. Create as many reservoirs and dams as possible to store rainwater.

This programme, which is restricted to the rural world, is an example of the practical forms that getting back to self-sufficiency might take.

And what about China? This question always comes up in discussions of de-growth. It is more unusual for someone to ask 'And what about India?' or 'What about Brazil?' It is clear that China's economic growth (and that of India) raises a global problem. China is on its way to becoming the planet's biggest polluter, even though it is far from being the biggest in relative terms. In 2004, its per capita ecological footprint corresponded to just one planet and was still six times smaller than that of the United States. (In the summer of 2007, China became the world's biggest source of greenhouse gases.) China is already the work-shop of the world. It would be immoral, and very difficult, to impose anything on the Chinese against their will. That the country's rising middle class (between 100 and 200 million people after all) should aspire to having their own cars and a share in the unbridled consumerism of the West is quite understandable, and all the less reprehensible in that we are largely responsible for it. Volkswagen and General Motors expect to be producing 3 million vehicles per year in China in years to come and Peugeot is investing on a huge scale so as not to be left behind. China does of course have its own car industry and supplies the home market (and to some extent the export market) by copying foreign marques. Whilst we can imagine what a happy society would look like, we ourselves have yet to enter a society that is both self-sufficient and sustainable, and, by definition frugal in material terms.

Be that as it may, the fate of the world and of humanity will largely be determined by the decisions taken by the Chinese leadership. The fact that they are aware of present ecological disasters and of the very real threats that hang over their future (and ours), and that they know that the ecological cost of growth will cancel out or exceed its benefits in terms of the ecological balance-sheet, together with an ancient tradition of wisdom that is far removed from the West's rationality and will to power, suggests that they will not rush into the blind alley that we find ourselves in, with almost no way out. According to the

Stern report (Stern 2006: 15), China has already adopted a vast programme to reduce the amount of energy used per unit of GDP by 20% between 2006 and 2010 and to promote the use of renewables. India is in a similar position and is preparing to implement a policy to improve energy efficiency over the same period.

A resolute commitment to a de-growth society that demonstrates that the 'model' is desirable and therefore exemplary is the best way to convince China, India and Brazil to change direction, to give them the means to do so and, in doing so, to save the planet from a terrible fate.

Is De-Growth Reformist or Revolutionary?

It is indeed a revolution. I should add, however, that, like Cornelius Castoriadis, I believe that 'revolution does not mean civil war or bloodshed'. That kind of violence seems all the less unavoidable in that, if André Gorz (1994 [1991]: 7) is to be believed (and Castoriadis would not have contradicted him in his last years), 'Capitalist civilization is moving inexorably towards catastrophic collapse. There is no longer any need for a revolutionary class to overthrow capitalism; it is digging its own grave, and that of industrial civilization in general.' That is just as well, as it is obvious that the triumph of capital has put an end to the class struggle. There are more losers than ever in this clash, which has lasted for centuries, but they are divided, destructured and decultured, and do not (or no longer) constitute a revolutionary class. Whilst the collapse of capitalism may be desirable, it by no means guarantees us a radiant future, and this is where revolution comes into its own. 'Revolution,' Castoriadis goes on (2005: 177),

> means that certain of society's central institutions will be changed thanks to the action of society itself: the explicit self-transformation of society condensed into a short space of time. . . . Revolution means that the majority of the

community enters a phase of *political* activity, or in other words *instituting* activity. The social imaginary gets to work and explicitly sets about transforming existing institutions.

In that sense, the de-growth society project is eminently revolutionary. We are taking about cultural change, as well as changes in the legal structure and relations of production. Whilst this is a political project, its implementation has more to do with an ethics of responsibility than with an ethics of conviction. Politics is not ethics, and politicians have to come to terms with the existence of evil. The quest for the common good is not a quest for the Good, but a quest for the lesser of two evils. And yet political realism does not mean surrendering to the banality of evil; it means containing evil within the bounds of the common good. In that sense, even radical and revolutionary politics can only be reformist, and must be reformist if it is not to drift into terrorism. The need for pragmatism in political action, which will be discussed in chapter 3, does not mean that we have to abandon the goals of our concrete utopia. Its revolutionary potential, and what José Bové (2007) aptly calls its fertility, are not incompatible with political reformism, provided that the inevitable compromises that have to be made at the practical level do not degenerate into compromises at the intellectual level.

– 3 –

A Political Programme

All those on the left who refuse to approach the question of growth without fairness in this way demonstrate that socialism is, in their view, nothing more than a continuation by other means of capitalist social relations and capitalist civilization, and of the bourgeois way of life and model of consumption.

(Gorz 1977)

Designing a coherent and desirable model for a de-growth society is not only a theoretical exercise but also a major step towards its political implementation. We have to further elaborate these concrete proposals, even though the in-depth self-transformation of society and its citizens seems to me to be more important than the outcome of any election. This does not necessarily mean that its birth will be spontaneous and painless. Politicians are now so concerned with mere politicking that they have little understanding of the realities that have to be changed and they cannot be trusted. That does not mean that there are no such things as electoral issues. In the best of cases, governments that wish to swim against the tide can do no more than decelerate, slow down and soften processes that are beyond their control. There is such a thing as a global 'cosmocracy' which, without taking any explicit decisions, is draining politics of its substance and imposing 'its' will through the 'dictatorship of the financial markets' (Duclos 1997). All governments are, whether they like it or not, capital's 'functionaries'.

The alternative to productivism exists at every level: individual, local, regional, national and global (special attention must be paid to the European level). But as the tyranny of the 'new masters of the universe' prefers to work at the higher levels, we must find the most pertinent levers if we are to be able to work in a concerted and complementary fashion.

Does the 'de-growth party' have an electoral programme? Is de-growth soluble in capitalism? Does the demand for it come from the right or from the left? Will the de-growth movement lead to the emergence of a new political programme? We will now try to answer these political questions.

An Electoral Programme

The virtuous circle of de-growth could be triggered by some very simple and apparently almost trivial measures.[1] The transition to a de-growth society can be described in a quasi-electoral programme that summarizes in a few points the 'common sense' implications of the above diagnosis.

For example:

1. *Get back to an ecological footprint equal to or smaller than a planet*, or in other words, other things being equal, to a material output equivalent to that of 1960–70.

---

[1] These do not preclude other public health measures, such as the introduction of a minimum wage, which has been proposed by MAUSS, or Jean-Paul Berlan's suggestion that all patents should simply be done away with. [MAUSS = Mouvement Anti-Utilitariste en Sciences Sociales (Anti-Utilitarian Movement in the Social Sciences) (Translator).]

How is it possible to reduce our ecological footprint by about 75% without going back to the Stone Age? Quite simply by making massive cuts in 'intermediate consumption', understood in the broad sense (transport, energy, packaging, advertising) without reducing the amount we ultimately consume. Getting back to the local level and eliminating waste would help.

2. Using the appropriate eco-taxes to *include transport costs* in the pollution caused by this activity.

The *a minima* external costs that are not borne by motorists reportedly amount to over 25 million euros per year in France, or to more than current domestic taxes on oil products (TIPP: *Taxe Intérieure sur les Produits Pétroliers*) (Rotillon 2006).

3. *Relocalize activities.* Given their harmful impact on the environment, we have to question the need to transport large numbers of people and large quantities of commodities around the world.

4. *Revitalize peasant agriculture*, or in other words do everything possible to encourage local, seasonal, natural and traditional agriculture.

We must gradually phase out the use of chemical pesticides that are allergenic. These include neurotoxins, products that depress the immune system, cause genetic mutations, cause cancer and that damage the endocrinal system and are reprotoxic, or capable of causing sterility (Nicolino and Veillerette 2007).

5. *Transform productivity gains into a reduction in working hours and job creation*, so long as unemployment persists.

Over the last two hundred years or so, hourly productivity has risen by a factor of 30 in France, whilst the number of hours worked by the average individual has fallen only by a factor of 2. The number of jobs has risen by a factor of 1.75, whilst production has risen by a factor of 26 (Marchand and Thélot 1977, cited Paquot 2006). We must invert our priorities thanks to job-sharing and an increase in leisure time.

6. *Encourage the 'production' of relational goods, such as friendship and neighbourliness*; my consumption of such goods does not reduce the available stock. On the contrary.

'Intellectual exchanges are basically different from commodity exchanges,' explains Bernard Maris (2006: 182).

> In an intellectual exchange, the giver does not lose anything and the receiver takes without dispossessing his or her interlocutor of anything. Knowledge, skills and art can therefore be shared and 'consumed' by everyone. Pythagoras's theorem is used by millions of individuals and applied to thousands of functions without anyone being deprived of it. Knowledge is a collective good, a fountain of youth from which we can all drink without causing others the least frustration.

'Happiness', Raoul Follereau used to say, 'is the only thing we can be sure of having once we have given it to someone.' All this 'enjoyment of the things we cannot buy':

> the pleasures of an animated conversation, a meal with friends, a good atmosphere at work, a town where we feel good, taking part in some form of cultural activity (professional activities, the arts, sport, etc.) and the whole range of relations with others in the broadest sense of the term. Most of these 'goods', and social life is their base par excellence, only exist if we enjoy them together. (Flahaut 2005: 151)

'Even the last Steppenwolf will agree', suggests Jean-Paul Besset (2005: 254), 'that most of the joys (and pains) of life are "relational".'

7. *Cut energy wastage* by a factor of 4 in accordance with the studies undertaken by the négaWatt association.[2]

8. *Heavy penalties for spending on advertising.* One might even adopt Nicolas Hulot's proposal as it stands:

> We have to look into the possibility of gradually introducing a complete ban on advertising in programmes aimed at children, and especially on adverts for products that are injurious to their health. The goal here is to restrict the extent to which viewers are conditioned to advertising at an age when they do not have the critical distance that is needed to resist its seductions. (Hulot 2006: 254)[3]

9. *Declare a moratorium on technoscientific innovation,* make a serious assessment of the situation and redirect scientific and technological research on the basis of new aspirations.[4]

We could, for example, develop 'green chemistry' rather than toxic molecules, environmental medicine rather than concentrating on genetics alone, and encourage research into agro-biology and agro-economics rather than into agro-industry (GM crops and other living pipe-dreams).

---

[2] The association brought together 100 experts and practitioners to study the possibility of cutting emissions of greenhouse gases in France by a factor of 4 by 2050 thanks to a combination of energy saving (cutting waste) and energy efficiency (reducing waste).

[3] For their part, the Greens' 2007 programme proposed a ban on advertising of public television channels (Canfin 2006: 112).

[4] The latter point echoes one of Cornelius Castoriadis's preoccupations (2005: 238): 'Where to draw the line? For the first time, in a non-religious society, we have to face the question: do we have to control the expansion of knowledge itself? And how can we do so without establishing an intellectual dictatorship? I think we can lay down a few basic principles: We do not want an exponential and unthinking rise in production; we want an economy that is a means and not the end of human life. We want knowledge to expand freely but . . . with *phronesis*.'

The moratorium should be extended to include big infrastructural projects (ITER, motorways, high-speed trains, incinerators, etc.).[5]

This platform, which was first outlined in an article published in *Le Monde diplomatique* in 2004, has a lot in common with subsequent proposals such as Nicolas Hulot's ecological contract and the 164 proposals put forward in the Appel de Paris (cf. Belpomme 2007). In both cases, we have a diagnosis of the threats and a prescription for a cure similar to my own, together with a wealth of information and details of concrete measures that are beyond our limited resources, and that in itself is cause for celebration. All this concurs with or complements most of the measures recommended by the ecologists: taxes upon machinery, the removal of taxes on work, land reform (creating new peasants) and efforts to encourage energy saving and cutting the consumption of natural resources.[6] Other possible measures include using high VAT-style taxes on the consumption of products whose relative prices continue to fall to finance a 'selected working hours' policy.

At the global level, we could adopt all these measures, and especially the fiscal measures proposed by Attac (Association for the Taxation of Financial Transactions to Aid Citizens) (2006):

- a tax on financial transactions: 'Introduce a tax on currency transactions and share dealing';
- an additional unitary tax on the profits of transnational firms to restrict tax dumping;

---

[5] 'It is imperative to establish an immediate moratorium on the building of new incinerators and the issue of new licences for coincineration' (Appel de Paris, cited Belpomme 2007: 257). [ITER is a joint international research and development project that aims to demonstrate the scientific and technical feasibility of fusion power (Translator).]

[6] See Fabrice Flipo's reply to Isaac Johsua: *http://decroissance.free.fr/ Reponse-Isaac_Johsua.rtf*.

- a global wealth tax: do away with tax havens and bank confidentiality;
- a tax on carbon emissions;
- a tax on highly active nuclear waste with a very long life.

To turn to the protection of the environment, global measures are unavoidable because pollution does not recognize frontiers. The problem of implementation is even more complex at this level, as action is for the moment taken, either directly or indirectly, at the state level.

This programme is centred on the internalization of external diseconomies (the damage caused by agents who leave the community to pick up the bill). All ecological and social dysfunctionalities – from road accidents to spending on anti-stress drugs – should and must be paid for by those who cause them. Eco-taxes are one way of making them do so. The three things that drive people to crime, denounced in chapter 1 – advertising, built-in obsolescence and credit – can be regarded as the growth society's negative externalities. Whilst their harmful effects cannot be measured, taxes and controls will make it possible to lessen their impact. This policy will have two effects: it will gradually reduce our ecological footprint, and it will give the community precious resources that will allow it to absorb their impact, to make the necessary investment in recycling, and to counter the inevitable dysfunctionalities caused by the current state of affairs. More could be done to improve public transport, for example, and to help the poorest members of society by imposing heavy tax increases on private transport.

Just imagine the environmental impact of internalizing the cost of spending on transport and health, or the impact that making firms pay for education, security and unemployment would have on the workings of our societies! In principle, these 'reformist' measures are in line with orthodox economic theory, as the liberal economist Cecil Pigou demonstrated in the early twentieth century.[7] Pigou demonstrated that, in order to achieve the best results (the greatest possible well-being for all consumers and producers), a system of taxes or subsidies must be used to correct prices. Taxes should ensure that the polluters bear the cost of the harmful external effects they have on their neighbours, and subsidies should be used to reward the producers of positive external effects. This was intended to encourage agents to take into account the social effects of their private decisions and to modify them accordingly. The principle of 'polluter pays' was born. 'It becomes possible to make private interests and the social (or general) interest to coincide without altering the actual mechanism of the market (which is something restrictive regulations cannot do) and simply by using a system of taxes to correct it' (Clerc 2006: 15). Nicolas Hulot's ecological pact is based upon the same principle. The difference is that, if these measures were taken to their ultimate conclusion, they would bring about a real revolution and would allow almost the entire programme for a de-growth society to be implemented. Firms that acted in accordance with the logic of capitalism would of course be discouraged and many activities would no longer be 'profitable'; the system would come to a halt. If, according to the International Center for Technological Assessment, invisible fuel costs were included – car accidents, air pollution, the cost of maintaining military bases to prevent the peoples of producer countries taking control of their own oil, subsidies to oil companies – the cost of petrol would soar from $1 a gallon to $14 (*Sierra Magazine*, March–April 2002: 15, cited Rasmussen 2004). With prices like that, civil aviation would come to a halt and there would probably not be many cars on the road.

---

[7] 'In a market economy, "externalities" are in theory internalized through taxation or the creation of property rights; market forces then lead to a situation that is preferable in social terms' (Aubertin and Viven 2006: 64).

Forcing firms to pay the full cost of the damage and risks they inflict on society would be another way of internalizing the negative externalities generated by the system. We already know that no insurance company is prepared to cover the risks inherent in the nuclear industry, climate change, GM crops or nanotechnologies.[8] One can imagine the paralysis that would result from compelling them to cover health risks, social risks (unemployment) or even aesthetic risks.

Any politician who proposed such a programme and implemented it when elected would be killed before the week was out. In December 1972, President Salvador Allende made an unusually lucid speech to the UN (Allende 1973). A few months later, he was assassinated because he had implemented a policy that was much less subversive than that outlined here. His explanation is more relevant than ever. He likened the tragedy of his country to that of a silent Vietnam. There were no troops occupying the country, and there were no planes flying over Chile. The country was, however, facing an economic blockade and had been denied credit by international financiers. It was facing a real battle between the multinationals and between states. States were no longer in control of their basic political, economic and military decisions because of the multinationals, which were not dependent on any state. They operated without taking any responsibility for their actions and were not controlled by any parliament or by any agency that represented the general interest. The political structure of the world had, in a word, been turned upside down. The big multinational companies were damaging the interests of the developing countries. Their oppressive and uncontrolled activities were also damaging the industrialized countries where they were based. And no one was even talking about 'globalization' in 1972.

[8] Insurance companies also refuse to cover the risks that might be generated by radiation from mobile phones.

The measures suggested here would bring us up against the real power of the plutocratic oligarchy that rules the world. Lobbies are its most obvious expression. Authorities, administrations and even research centres are all to a greater or lesser extent controlled by what is now a global complex. It should be recalled that many of the alarm bells sounded by scientists (asbestos, aflotoxin, fiprolnil and imidacloine, heparine, electromagnetic fields, dioxin and chemicals affecting the endocrinal system . . .) have been silenced by government agencies because of the pressure of economic interests. The laboratories concerned have lost their funding and in some cases scientists have been removed from their posts (sometimes with the collusion of unions trying to 'protect' jobs) (Cicolella and Benoît-Browaeys 2005).

A programme for a national policy of de-growth seems paradoxical. The implementation of realistic and rational proposals has little chance of being adopted and still less chance of succeeding unless the entire system is subverted. Its subversion presupposes a change in the imaginary, and the only thing that can bring that about is the realization of the fertile utopia of a convivial and autonomous society.

There is, then, no shortage of proposals or solutions, but the preconditions for their implementation are not there. There are several possible scenarios for a gentle transition and very gradual measures could begin to implement the cuts that are needed. The important point is that a radical change of direction is needed. We therefore have to create the preconditions for that change of direction. The goal of a more sophisticated project is of course to create those preconditions.

Jobs for All in a De-Growth Society

The harshest criticism from de-growth's opponents 'on the left' has to do with the abandonment of full employment implicit in our project.[9] When we are asked to be 'realistic' in this context, what solutions do those who object to continued growth – they have been described as the 'kids of the rich' by a journalist on *Le Monde* – have to offer to the problem of unemployment?[10]

They argue that using consumption, and therefore growth, to relaunch the economy has to be ruled out. A sharp reduction in the number of hours we have to work is therefore a necessary precondition for getting away from the work-based model for growth, but also for ensuring that everyone has a satisfying job; that will bring about the two-thirds reduction in the consumption of natural resources that is required in France. Hence the apparent discrepancy, in terms of realism and time-scale, between our proposals and those of the 'relaunchers': we will not immediately ban the heavy goods vehicles that transport consumer goods we do not need (as well as most of those we do need) or cut the number of cars on the road or planes in the air. It will take time to relocalize production, trade and ways of life. That is a challenge because we urgently need a political ecology, even if it means upsetting the political ant's nest. This is not a long-term issue. We must start today, think in terms of stages and not lose sight of our goal. And besides, and whatever our detractors may think, ecological politics is not incompatible with social policy. Indeed, it is a precondition for any change that does not just plaster over the cracks. 'We cannot solve the environmental crisis without solving social problems,' Murray Bookchin said in 1990. That may well be true, but the converse may be even truer: we

---

[9] 'Jean-Maries Harribey basically criticizes us for four things', Paul Ariès rightly notes (2005: 87): 'contraction without abandoning capitalism, unrestricted contraction, a failure to see that capitalism is not the only possible economy, and an abandonment of the possibility of full employment.'

[10] 'The doctrine of de-growth has to be seen for what it is: a hare-brained idea dreamed up by the completely selfish kids of the rich' (Pierre-Antoine Delhommais, *Le Monde*, 30 July 2006).

cannot resolve social problems without resolving the environmental crisis.

When it comes to jobs, some opponents of growth refer to 'our ancestors who, in order to survive, worked hard and were reduced to drudgery'. They even think that, far from creating unemployment, de-growth will require us to work longer hours and will create a job surplus (Cheynet and Cheynet 2004).[11] An end to productivism and the exploitation of workers in the South would generate more work in order to satisfy the equivalent level of final consumption (which could be achieved be greatly reducing intermediate consumption).[12] According to a study from the organic Fédération nationale des agriculteurs, 90,000 jobs could be created in France if the number of organic farmers rose from today's wretched 2% to Austria's 9%. If that figure rose to 15%, between 120,000 and 150,000 jobs could be created (Canfin 2006: 107). We will also have to create more jobs when the oil runs out. Fossil fuels (oil and natural gas) now provide 80% of the world's supply of primary energy. As a barrel of oil contains the energy equivalent of 25,000 hours of human labour (or, to be more accurate, 10,000 hours, given the efficiency of the engines that are best at converting fuel into mechanical labour), our daily consumption of hydrocarbons is equivalent to the work of over three hundred billion human

---

[11] This reference to the past is problematic: which ancestors are they talking about? Our Stone Age ancestors 'worked' for no more than three to four hours a week to ensure the survival of the group, as Marshall Sahlins demonstrates in his famous *Stone-Age Economics* (1972). Without going quite so far back in time, Gorz argues (1994 [1991]: 110) that one thousand hours per year was the norm until the beginning of the eighteenth century. Now, one thousand hours per year works out at an average of twenty hours a week, or in other words much the same as the not exactly furious pace of the Neolithic.

[12] According to the Fédération nationale de l'agriculture biologique's Dominque Vérot, organic farming would require a work force 30% per hectare greater than that used by traditional farming, but productivity would fall by about 50%. Hence the need for a 250% rise in the workforce (Sas 2006: 188).

beings: 'It is as though everyone on earth had fifty slaves at their disposal' (Cochet 2005: 192, 139).[13]

If France applied the European directive and produced 20% of its electricity from renewable sources such as solar and wind power, 240,00 jobs could be created (Canfin 2006: 19). A document published by the European Commission in 2005 shows that every one million euros invested in energy efficiency creates 16 full-time jobs, as opposed to the 4.5 created by a nuclear power station and the 4.1 created by a coal-fired plant. In other words, it costs twice as much to produce one kilowatt-hour as it does to save it.

We have, therefore, four factors with different effects: (1) the undeniable loss of productivity that would result from the abandoning of the thermo-industrial model, polluting technologies and energy-greedy plant; (2) the relocalization of activities and a halt to the exploitation of the South; (3) the creation of green jobs in new sectors of activity; and (4) a change in our way of life and the removal of useless *needs* (major cutbacks in advertising, tourism, transport, the car industry, agribusiness, biotechnologies, etc.). The first three have the effect of increasing the quantity of labour, whilst the fourth has the opposite effect. The 'reserve supply' is so great that the needs of a convivial *art de vivre* for all could be met by a considerable reduction in the number of hours we have to work. For centuries, productivity gains have been systematically transformed into greater output rather than into reducing the effort required. It should also be recalled that productivity gains from technological innovations are systematically over-stated because their less visible costs are not taken into account. At the same time, the potential

---

[13] 'The average petrol engine can transform the 10,000 kcal contained in a litre of fuel into the 2.3 kWh of mechanical energy required to drive the turn-pin of a cement mixer or the crankshaft of a car; that figure is equivalent to more than four days ordinary muscular effort on the part of a human being' (Cochet 2005: 91).

productivity gains from convivial tools are systematically under-stated.[14] It is reasonable to conclude that, after the sudden fall in overall productivity that would result from the abandonment of toxic technologies, we could expect modest but steady productivity gains, especially in terms of eco-efficiency. That would, at least in theory, allow a gentle transition. Different simulation models can of course be developed and discussed. A de-growth society could, at all events, provide productive waged work for all those who want it rather than, by more or less artificial means, transforming non-market activities into waged labour and increasing the number of parasitic or servile jobs.

It is also possible that, in its early stages, a de-growth policy would have the paradoxical effect, at the macroeconomic level, of increasing output by targeting both the demand for ecological products and appliances and the trades needed to produce them.

Lester Brown (2001) has demonstrated that nine productive sectors would have to be developed in a 'solar' economy, or in other words one based upon renewables: the construction of wind turbines, the production of photovoltaic cells, the bicycle industry, the production of hydrogen and the appropriate engines, building light railways, organic farming and reforestation. New trades must be developed at every level from forestry to eco-architecture.

The cuts, repairs and recycling that would result from the abandonment of built-in obsolescence will also give rise to new activities that would be very different from those proposed by the official anti-liberals of the traditional left who want to build hospitals and schools in order to *save* jobs. I am not suggesting a general but unfocused relaunch of the economy. The main enemy is over-consumption or hyper-consumption, and not economic

---

[14] 'By applying a well-calibrated ball-bearing between two neolithic millstones, a man could now grind in a day what took his ancestors a week' (Illich 1974: 71).

contraction. De-growth is not a rigid dogma but it does challenge the logic of growth for growth's sake. As well as reducing working hours and the number of harmful activities, the expansion of new and desirable activities could therefore have a positive outcome in terms of jobs.

It is difficult to predict how long the transition will take, but productivity gains could be translated into cuts in working hours and job creation without any detrimental effects on wages (or at least the lowest wages) or final output, though its content would have to be transformed. The transition can be painless, but the important thing is that there must be no compromise as to its objectives. If we change our lives, we can solve the problem of unemployment, but if we focus on the problem of jobs for the sake of jobs there is a danger that we will never change society and that we will head straight for disaster.

De-Growth: Beyond the Work-Based Society

A dramatic reduction in working hours is a first defence against flexibility and job insecurity. The right to work, which the neo-liberals oppose because it is a source of rigidity, must therefore be preserved and strengthened. It can only encourage the de-growth we need. Decent minimum wage thresholds have to be defended against the economist's theory of voluntary unemployment, which is a sham. Getting back to the 'decommodification' of work is an imperative. The current emphasis on the 'lowest social bid' is as unacceptable as that of the 'lowest ecological bid'.[15] In 1946, a 20-year-old wage-earner could expect to spend one third of his waking life at work. In 1975, he could expect to spend one quarter of it at work, and

---

[15] On this point, the reader is referred to my comments in *Justice sans limites* (Latouche 2003a), especially in chapter 6.

today's equivalent figure is one fifth. Does he therefore feel that he has been set free from work? Probably less so than ever before. 'For wage-earners,' notes Bernard Maris (2006: 109), 'this is not the end of work, as the underlying reduction in the number of hours worked would appear to show, but work without end, job insecurity, isolation, stress, fear and the certainty that they will have to leave their workplace quite quickly.'

Reducing working hours and changing the content of work are therefore primarily social choices resulting from the cultural revolution brought about by de-growth. Giving citizens more unconstrained time in order to allow them to blossom in their political, private and artistic lives, and play or contemplation, is the precondition for developing a new form of wealth. 'Our talents will take the place in our hearts that needs have taken away; our artistic, poetic and scientific talents will multiply and put down roots day by day' (Tarde 1980 [1896]: 92).

The basic question is therefore not the precise number of hours we need to work, but work's role as a social 'value'. We have lost our bearings in recent years, and that has been of some concern to the professional politicians of the left. Some prophesy the end or metamorphosis of work (Gorz 1994 [1991]; Méda 1995; Rifkin 1995; Robin 1994), whilst others have revived the ideology of work in a surrealist fashion. The same uncertainty surrounds retirement age; whereas early retirement used to be in fashion, there is now a tendency to argue that we should work longer.[16] Some argue that the RMI[17] must lead to a new Speenhamland, and both the left and the right are demand-

[16] According to Wim Kok's 2003 report on the enlargement of the European Union, working after the age of sixty must become the norm (Ramaux 2006: 89).

[17] The RMI, which is equivalent to half the SMIC (*salaire minimum interprofessionel de croissance*), is paid to unemployed active members of society who are looking for work. Speenhamland refers to the birthplace of the system of subsidies given to poor workers in England until 1930. It was deemed to be counter-productive.

ing a 'citizen income', whilst the 'thirty-five-hour week' has come under direct attack. French society, like all Western societies, is totally confused about the issue of work.

De-growth, in contrast, implies both a quantitative reduction in working hours and the qualitative transformation of work. Certain individuals have already succeeded in escaping from the growth society, and their experiences may show us a way forward, provided that we can resist the spiral of exponential accumulation and escape the infernal cycle of needs and income. This is the logic behind REPAS (Réseau d'échange des pratiques alternatives et solidaires; see Barras 2002; Lulek 2003). Working less and in different ways may mean rediscovering a taste for leisure or recovering the lost abundance of the hunter-gatherer societies analysed by Marshall Sahlins (1972). Limiting one's own needs is one way of becoming an 'objector to growth'. Doing so realizes the objective preconditions for the changes at the social level that must be one of the goals of building a de-growth society.

'Changing life' (the Socialist slogan in 1981) or working 'towards a different world' (Attac's slogan in 2002) can be done today, but not with old recipes and not without making a break with the past. Possible compromises over how we make the transition must not make us lose sight of our objectives, which are not negotiable. The relative failure of the 'thirty-five-hour week' resulted from that lack of determination. Looking at the reasons for the failure of the German SPD's (Social Democratic Party) 1989 programme is just as instructive (Gorz 1994 [1991]: 28): it called for 'The reduction of weekly working hours to thirty spread over five days, to which would also be added the right to a sabbatical year and additional (paid) holidays for the parents of young children and those in need of care – i.e. an average working live of around a thousand years.' It further openly advocated de-growth: 'Those activities which threaten the natural foundations of life must diminish and disappear' (cited Gorz 1994 [1991]:

32).[18] Such activities include the nuclear industry and, to some extent, the use of private cars. The programme was based on the idea that ecological rationality and economic (capitalist) rationality could be reconciled by the famous win-win strategies (Gorz 1994 [1991]: 33): 'In the long term, what is ecologically unreasonable cannot be economically rational . . . Ecological necessities have to become the basic principles of economic activity. If we set about ecological modernization in time, we shall improve our chances of conquering tomorrow's markets and improve the competitiveness of our economy.' This reluctance to challenge the logic of capitalism probably explains the failure of the SPD (Gorz 1994 [1991]: 31):

> It would be an illusion to believe – and paradoxical to hope – that ecological rationalization can compensate for the decline and conversion of the classical industries by employing in an 'environmental economy' the labour and capital that are saved elsewhere. For a great many enterprises, ecological conversion can be an engine of growth during the transitional period, but this cannot be the goal from the macro-economic point of view. . . . This is a policy for which there is no alternative, and one which must not be presented as an option motivated by the economic opportunities it affords.

Ultimately, and apart from a few remarkable advances at the ecological level in Germany and some social gains in France (the RMI and the thirty-five-hour week), neither social Europe nor ecological Europe has begun to achieve anything, even though most of its governments are on the left.

The content of this 'freeing time' policy has yet to be specified. In 1962, the sociologist Joffre Dumazedier pub-

---

[18] However, 'those activities must grow which secure the basic element of life and improve its quality, [which] promote self-determination and autonomous creative activities' (cited Gorz 1994 [1991]: 32).

lished his pioneering study *Towards a Society of Leisure* (Dumazedier 1967 [1962]). In it, he examined in detail the three functions of leisure: relaxation, entertainment and (personal) development. His whole construct is based upon the hypothesis of an 'autonomous subject'. At about the same time, Henri Lefebvre was demonstrating that: 'We no longer create ourselves through, by and with work. . . . In the guided bureaucratic consumer society . . . the meaning of life is a life devoid of meaning' (cited Paquot 2005: 29).

Unless life is 're-enchanted', the de-growth project, too, is doomed to failure. We still need to give liberated time a meaning. So long as waged work has not been transformed, the working classes will have no 'capacity for leisure', that is to say, 'the objective and subjective means for occupying the time freed up by autonomous activities' (Rainer Land, cited Gorz 1994 [1991]: 58). As Daniel Mothé (1977) has demonstrated, under present conditions, time that has been liberated from work has not necessarily been liberated from the economy. Most of our free time does not lead to a reappropriation of life and does not represent an escape from the dominant market model. Time is still often devoted to activities that have been commodified, and those activities do not allow consumers to become the producers of their own lives. They are shunted on to a parallel track. Free time is becoming more and more professionalized and industrialized. Escaping the present productivist, work-based system presupposes a very different form of organization in which leisure and play are as highly valued as work, and in which social relations take priority over the production and consumption of throwaway products that are useless or even harmful. 'Basically,' writes François Brune (2006), 'we are faced with the reconquest of personal time. A qualitative time. A time that cultivates slowness and contemplation because it has been set free from thinking about products.' To rephrase Hannah Arendt, it is not only that the two repressed components of the *vita activa* – the work of the artist or artisan and political activity in the true sense – will be restored to the same dignity as labour; the *vita contemplativa* itself will be rehabilitated. According to André Gorz (1994 [1991]: 61), we need 'a *politics* of time which embraces the reshaping of the urban and natural environment, cultural politics, education and training, and perhaps the social services and public amenities in such a way as to create more scope for self-managed activities, mutual aid, voluntary cooperation and production for one's own use'.

It is, perhaps, here that the difference between our 'sensibilities' and those of our critics is most obvious. Saving jobs at all cost, as recommended by Christophe Ramaux and, in more nuanced terms, Jean-Marie Harribey, is usually an expression, conscious or otherwise, of a visceral attachment to the work-based society. And the point is to escape it, not to save it. Pro-work propaganda has been so successful that its victims have updated it by redefining 'real' work as a creative activity that can be likened to the 'labour' of giving birth, and thus breaking the historical link between work and the wage-system.[19] They even bemoan the fact that work has not extended its empire and its hold on life, and that house 'work' and charity work are not taken into account or remunerated.

Thanks to the alchemy of the market, the economy has often proved itself capable of creating more jobs and actually increasing monetary values, but that has not led to increased satisfaction and may even have reduced satisfaction. Factoring in the cost of transport, packaging, advertising and branding can increase the price of a pharmaceutical molecule, yoghurt, water or any foodstuff but it does

[19] Some try desperately to 'save work' by redefining it in ideal terms and forgetting about 'actual existing work'. That is Alain Soupiot's position. It is no accident that this argument was used against me in a debate with the Greens 'to save development'. This is in fact all part of the same struggle, and the issues are the same (see Méda 2001).

nothing to increase their effectiveness.[20] Yet this artificial increase in value consumes large quantities of energy (transport) and various raw materials (packaging, canning, advertising . . .), and any attempt to reduce growth has to prioritize the reduction of this intermediate consumption. The almost desperate attempts that are being made to increase market values still more on an exhausted planet (examples include fish farming, GM crops and nuclear energy) have had a truly catastrophic ecological impact. They certainly create jobs (which are often badly paid), but we could obtain the same ultimate satisfaction by drastically cutting the working week and greatly reducing our ecological footprint.

'By dint of monetizing, professionalizing and transforming into jobs the few remaining production and service activities we still perform for ourselves, might we not reduce our ability to look after ourselves almost to the point where it disappears, thus undermining the foundations of existential autonomy, not to mention the foundations of lived sociality and the fabric of human relationships?' asks André Gorz (1994 [1991]: 51–2). The various tricks that are used to convert activities into work on the pretext of saving jobs are very similar to those used to count the jobless and to remove them from the unemployment statistics. 'There might,' Gorz adds (1994 [1991]: 47), 'be no limits to the development of employment if it were possible to transform into acts of paid work those activities which people have hitherto performed for themselves.' As he notes (1994 [1991]: 50–1): 'In other words, from now on, job creation depends mainly not on *economic* activity, not

[20] Bertrand de Jouvenel reports (2002 [1968]: 178) that 'In the United States, per capita consumption of food, measured in constant prices, reportedly rose by 75% between 1909 and 1957. The Department of Agriculture calculates that the rise of physiological consumption was at most between 12 and 15%. According to Kuzenets's analysis, at least four-fifths of this apparent increase was, in other words, a reflection of the growth of the transport and distribution services relating to foodstuffs.'

on the *productive* substitution of waged work for individuals' private production but on its *counter-productive* substitution.' It creates, in other words, a new servant class or a new serfdom. Hence the ambiguity of all the 'personal services' we keep hearing about.

Conversely, rediscovering quality outside the logic of the market reduces economic values. This becomes quite obvious if production ceases to be dominated by the market: we both reduce our ecological footprint and GDP and at the same time increase a certain form of personal satisfaction. That is why the demand of some anti-globalization campaigners (create more service sector jobs to cut unemployment) is a bad good idea.[21]

Gaining more 'free' time is an essential precondition for the decolonization of the economy. It concerns workers and wage-earners, but also stressed middle managers, bosses who are harassed by the competition and members of the liberal professions who are caught in the vice of compulsive growth. Far from being our adversaries, they can become our allies as we build a de-growth society.

Is De-Growth Soluble in Capitalism?

Can we have de-growth under capitalism? This question comes up in practically every public debate. Some critics accuse us of coming to terms with capitalist exploitation because we denounce globalization and growth without always explicitly describing them as ultraliberal and capitalist.[22] We are in fact being criticized for throwing the baby of development, growth and the economy out with

---

[21] Attali and Champain (2005) have turned stating the obvious into an art form: 'Regarding job-seeking as an activity would be enough to do away with unemployment.' As Christophe Ramaux (2006) remarks, 'Someone had to come up with that bright idea.'

[22] This is the first of the four criticisms addressed to de-growth by Jean-Marie Harribery (2004).

the dirty water of capitalism and neo-liberalism. We refuse, in other words, to 'save' the fantasy of an *alternative* economy, an *alternative* growth and an *alternative* development (which can variously be described as Keynesian, public, socialist, human, sustainable, clean . . .).

The traditional response from a certain section of the left consists in seeing the entity known as 'capitalism' as the source of all problems and all our powerlessness and, therefore, defining it as the citadel we have to demolish. Giving the enemy a face is in fact now problematic, as economic entities, like the transnational firms that actually hold power, are, by their very nature, incapable of exerting their power directly. On the one hand, Big Brother is anonymous; on the other, the servitude of his subjects is more *voluntary* than ever because their manipulation of commercial advertising is infinitely more insidious than that of political propaganda. How, under these conditions, can we 'politically' challenge the megamachine?

We do not dwell on a specific critique of capitalism because it seems to us that there is no point in stating the obvious. That critique was, for the most part, put forward by Karl Marx. And yet a critique of capitalism is not enough: we also need a critique of any growth society. And that is precisely what Marx fails to provide. A critique of the growth society implies a critique of capitalism, but the converse is not necessarily true. Capitalism, neo-liberal or otherwise, and productivist socialism are both variants on the same project for a growth society based upon the development of the productive forces, which will supposedly facilitate humanity's march in the direction of progress.

Because it cannot integrate ecological constraints, the Marxist critique of modernity remains terribly ambiguous. The capitalist economy is criticized and denounced, but the growth of the forces it unleashes is described as 'productive' (even though they are as destructive as they are productive). Ultimately, growth, seen in terms of the production/jobs/consumption trio, is credited with every, or almost every, virtue, even though, when seen in terms of the accumulation of capital, it is held responsible for every scourge: the proletarianization of workers, their exploitation and impoverishment, not to mention imperialism, wars, crises (including, of course, ecological crises), and so on. Changing the relations of production (and this is what the revolution we both need and want means) is therefore reduced to meaning a more or less violent revolution in the status of those who have a right to a share in the fruits of growth. We can quibble about its content, but the principle remains unchallenged.

Given that the growth and development in question mean, respectively, the growth of the accumulation of capital and the development of capitalism, de-growth can only mean the contraction of accumulation, capitalism, exploitation and predation. The point is not just to slow accumulation down but to challenge the concept of accumulation itself so as to reverse the destructive process.[23]

We obviously cannot expect the non-Marxist left to raise this problem, as it came to an understanding with the system long ago.

Our conception of the de-growth society means neither an impossible return to the past nor a compromise with capitalism. It means going beyond modernity (thanks, if possible, to an orderly transition). 'Capitalism can no more be "persuaded" to limit growth than a human being can be "persuaded" to stop breathing' (Murray Bookchin,

---

[23] It is regrettable, and perhaps tragic, that the relationship between Karl Marx and Sergei Podolinsky came to nothing. Podolinsky (1850–91), a Ukrainian aristocrat and scientist exiled in France, was a brilliant forerunner of political ecology who attempted to reconcile socialist thought with the second law of thermodynamics, and to synthesize Marx, Darwin and Carnot. It is in any case likely that, had the intellectual encounter taken place, we could have avoided many of socialism's blind alleys, not to mention a few polemics over whether or not de-growth was a leftist or rightist policy (see Martinez-Alier and Naredo 1982).

cited Martin 2006). De-growth is fundamentally anti-capitalist. Not so much because it denounces the contradictions and ecological and social limitations of capitalism as because it challenges its 'spirit', in the sense that Max Weber sees the 'spirit of capitalism' as a precondition for its existence. Whilst it is, in the abstract, possible to conceive of an economy that is ecologically compatible with the continued existence of a capitalism of the immaterial, that prospect is unrealistic when it comes to the imaginary foundations of a market society, namely excess and unbridled (pseudo-)domination. A generalized capitalism cannot but destroy the planet in the same way that it is destroying society and anything else that is collective.

'Beyond capitalism'. This is a convenient way of describing a historical process that is anything but simple: eliminating capitalists, outlawing the private ownership of the means of production, and abolishing the wage relationship or doing away with money. Doing so would plunge society into chaos, and could not be done without using terror on a vast scale. And it would not be enough to abolish the capitalist imaginary. On the contrary.

Can we still talk of money, markets, profits and the wage system in a post-development society?[24] These institutions, which some are too quick to identify with capitalism itself, are not necessarily obstacles in themselves. Many human societies are familiar with markets (especially in Africa), currencies and commercial, financial and even industrial profits (though it would be more accurate to describe them as 'industrious', as we are talking about artisans). They are also familiar with paid labour that takes the form of what we call the wage system. And yet those 'economic' relations do not dominate either the production or circulation of 'goods and services'. What is more important, they are not so articulated as to form a system. They are neither market societies, wage-based

---

[24] I discuss this at some length in the final part of my *Justice sans limites* (Latouche 2003a).

societies nor industrial societies, and still less are they capitalist societies, even though both *capital* and *capitalists* can be found in them. The imaginary of these societies has been colonized by the economy to such a minor extent that they do not realize that they have an economy. Getting beyond development, the economy and growth therefore does not imply abandoning all the social institutions that the economy has annexed; it means *embedding them* in a different logic.[25] De-growth can be regarded as en 'eco-socialism', especially if we agree with Gorz (1994 [1991]: 30) that socialism is 'the positive response to the disintegration of social bonds ensuing from the commodity and competitive relations characteristic of capitalism'.

Is De-Growth a Right-Wing Policy or a Left-Wing Policy?

The de-growth movement is revolutionary and anti-capitalist (and even anti-utilitarian) and its programme is basically political. But is it a left-wing policy or a right-wing policy? Many ecologists agree with Thierry Pacquot

---

[25] On this point, I agree with Cornelius Castoriadis's analysis: 'Marxism implies the absurd idea that the market as such and commodities as such "personify" alienation; to say so is absurd because relations between human beings in an extended society cannot be "personal" in the way that they can be inside a family. They are always socially mediated, and always will be. In the context of a society that is developed to even a minimal extent, that mediation is known as the *market* (exchange)' (Castoriadis 2005: 190). He goes on: 'It is perfectly obvious to me: a complex society cannot exist without impersonal means of exchange. Money fulfils that function, and in that respect it is very important. It is one thing to take away one of its functions in capitalist and precapitalist economies: that of serving as an instrument for the individual accumulation of wealth and the acquisition of the means of production. But to the extent that money is a unit of value and a means of exchange, money is a great invention and one of humanity's great creations' (2005: 198).

(2006: 113) that 'the real political duality is no longer that between "right" and "left", but that between those who care about ecology and the predators'. That is probably true, and it could be argued that the programme we are outlining – and it is primarily a matter of common sense – has as few supporters on the left as it does on the right. And yet those partisans who are not 'on the left' (Nicolas Hulot, Corinne Lepages, Yann Arthus-Bertrand) are often strangely silent when it comes to the predators.

It is true that there is such a thing as a right-wing critique of modernity, just as there is such a thing as a right-wing anti-utilitarianism and a right-wing anti-capitalism (although it is poorly represented in the parliamentary right). It is not surprising to find that right-wing critics of the ideology of work and anti-productivism use the same arguments as us. It has to be admitted that despite Paul Lafargue's fine *The Right to be Lazy* (Lafargue 1907) – Lafargue was Marx's son-in-law – which is still one of the harshest attacks on the ideology of work and productivism, and despite the anarchist tradition within Marxism that was revived by the Frankfurt School, the workers' council movement and situationism, radical critiques of modernity are more highly developed on the right than on the left. Hannah Arendt and Cornelius Castoriadis did a lot to develop such critiques, which have also been influenced by the arguments of counter-revolutionary thinkers like Edmund Burke, Louis de Bonald or Joseph de Maistre, but they remain marginal in political terms. Maoism, Trotskyism and other forms of leftism are just as productivist as the orthodox communisms.

There are, however, no grounds for confusing right- and left-wing anti-productivism, anti-capitalism or anti-utilitarianism.

Even though left-wing governments adopt right-wing policies and, because they do not dare to 'decolonize the imaginary', condemn themselves to social liberalism, those who object to growth and want to build a de-growth society that is convivial, peaceful and sustainable can tell the difference (minimal as it may be) between Jospin and Chirac, Royal and Sarkozy, Schröder and Merkel, Prodi and Berlusconi, or even Blair and Thatcher. When they cast their votes (and we advise them to do so), they know that, even though no government programme takes into account the need to reduce our ecological footprint, they still have to look towards the values of sharing, solidarity, equality and fraternity rather than those of the freedom to do business (and to exploit). If, like Hans Jonas, we extend those values to future generations, we have to put an end to the pillaging of nature, if not the massacre of other species, and get away from a narrow anthropocentrism. That is why we have to be resolute in the fight against globalization and economic neo-liberalism.

A *contrario*, writes Hervé Kempf (2007: 114), 'the cunning of history seems to mean that authoritarian governments use ecological necessity as a way of justifying restrictions of freedom without doing anything about inequality. Managing epidemics, nuclear accidents, pollution peaks and climate change could all be invoked as reasons for restricting our liberties.' We could easily move from the rampant totalitarianism of our current plutocratic oligarchy, which still preserves a semblance of formal democracy, to a muscular eco-fascism or eco-totalitarianism. André Gorz (1994 [1991]: 43–4) outlines how this could happen:

> The reproduction of the 'natural' base of life can itself be industrialized and developed as a profitable eco-business, obeying the same imperatives of profitability as other consumer goods industries. . . . An ecological techno-fascism would also be capable of reproducing the bases of life, by artificially replacing natural cycles, turning nature into business . . . and so industrializing the reproduction of life, even of human life, commodifying foetuses and organs and instrumentalizing genetic stock, including that of humans, in accordance with the demands of productivity and profit maximization.

Do We Need a De-Growth Party?

'In the event of a world-wide ecological disaster, for example, one can easily imagine authoritarian regimes introducing draconian restrictions on a panicked and apathetic population. . . . And if there is no new movement and no reawakening of the democratic project, "ecology" could very well be integrated into a neo-fascist ideology' (Castoriadis 2005: 246). If we react to that terrifying prospect by gambling on de-growth, we must assume that the attractions of a convivial utopia, together with the need for change, will encourage a 'decolonization of the imaginary' and will do enough to encourage 'virtuous' behaviours that will help us to find a reasonable solution. Castoriadis's analysis reaches the same conclusion: 'It is essential to insert the ecological component into a radical democratic political programme. And the imperative to do so is all the greater in that the challenge to the values and orientations of contemporary society, which is implicit in such a project, is indissociable from the critique of the imaginary of "development" on which we are living' (Castoriadis 2005: 246).

Does this necessarily mean that we now have to reify the movement in the form of a de-growth party? I think not. There is a danger that the premature institutionalization of the de-growth programme in the form of a political party would lead us into the trap of mere politicking. When that happens, political actors become divorced from social realities and trapped within the political game. The preconditions that might allow us to dream of building a de-growth society have yet to be established, and it is doubtful that such a society would be built within the outdated framework of the nation-state (see Fotopoulos 2001; Latouche 2005d). And yet politicking seems to exercise a growing seduction as its impotence becomes more and more pathetic, and candidates are queuing up to capitalize as quickly as possible on the (very relative) success of this or that legitimate demand. I think, on the contrary, that it is more important to influence the debate, to persuade people to take certain arguments into consideration, and to help to change attitudes. That is now our mission and our ambition.

Conclusion

Is De-Growth a Humanism?

Have men gone mad? I think so, and I am becoming more
and more convinced that they have. All this can and will
lead only to our destruction. Unless . . .

(Belpomme 2007: 56)

Like all ecologists, advocates of de-growth are suspected
of rejecting the anthropocentrism of the Enlightenment
tradition in favour of an unwavering ecocentrism and,
therefore, of supporting a form of deep ecology that takes
an 'anti-speciesist' stance. They are, in other words, suspected of seeing the survival of cockroaches as more
important than that of human beings. Those who introduce a spiritual, or even religious, dimension are immediately accused of *ecolatry*. Then comes the accusation that
they are calling for a return to a local or closed communitarianism. And then the invectives start: they are retro-
grade, obscurantist and reactionary (see, for instance,
Jacob 2006).

As they do not subscribe to a superficial view of ecology,
the advocates of de-growth are supposedly believers in
'deep' ecology. Deep ecology, or at least the form of deep
ecology popularized by Arne Naess, does, perhaps, go too
far in the direction of ecocentrism, but many of those who

argue the case against continued growth claim to be humanists. This issue is surrounded by a lot of confusion, and the tendency to argue in Manichaean terms does little to dispel it.[1] Do we really have to choose between ecocentrism and anthropocentrism, humanism and anti-speciesism, absolute relativism and dogmatic universalism, and modernity and tradition? How can we get away from these old debates, which are interconnected and recurrent, and which, ultimately, can never be decided one way or the other? Does rejecting the humanism of George W. Bush, the anthropocentrism of Descartes, Bacon and Teilhard de Chardin and the racist universalism of Kant[2] necessarily mean that we have to reject human specificity, fail to recognize human dignity and trap ourselves into cultural ghettoes?

We must, first of all, be agreed as to what humanism is. It is basically the belief that the concept of a 'human being' implies an essential/substantial essence that transcends the mere existence of the species. The humanity of human beings, in other words, exists independently of the concrete existence of concrete human beings (past, present and future) as an 'abstraction' and not as a 'common denominator'. The human essence derives, it is claimed, from something that makes humans radically different from other species. Some call it the soul, and others reason. That transcendence is not only immanent in the generality idea of 'man', but inscribed within a problematic conceptual

---

[1] Alexandre Adler provides an almost caricatural example in his article on 'The Return of the Nihilist Revolution' (*Le Monde*, 24 April 1999). He contrasts 'universal forces, such as trade, technology, law, democracy and the advancement of women' with 'a common programme that really is anti-globalization, anti-humanist and anti-liberal . . . that is being brewed up in the retorts of a new authoritarian populism on a global scale'.

[2] 'The explicit racism and anti-Semitism of Kant and most of his intellectual brothers in Western Europe have their sources in the field of the logical immanence that is characteristic of the enlightenment subject' (Kurz 2006: 36–7). On Teilhard de Chardin, see Flipo (2007: 201).

eternity. Humans are therefore superior beings who have (natural) rights over other species and over nature. These are human rights or the rights of man. Hence the importance of the sixteenth-century Valladolid controversy over whether or not Indians had souls (at the same time, the said Indians were leaving white prisoners to rot in water to see if they really were extraterritorial entities such as gods, ancestors or demons . . .). 'Humanism, which puts man at the centre of the universe, can be defined as an *anthropocentrist* particularism' (Kessous 2006: 54).

There is no doubt that this is true in the case of Westerners (and therefore in my own case, given that I am a Westerner). That is why we resist, and must resist, all forms of racism and discrimination (skin colour, sex, religion, ethnicity . . .). Unfortunately, they are all too common in the West, even today. Think of Guantánamo Bay, Abu Ghraib, the Sarkozy laws or the wall along the US–Mexican border. The American legislation that legalized torture reached one of the most repulsive peaks of hypocrisy on the part of Christian humanists who claim to be the defenders of democracy and human rights. The problem is that, for very many cultures, the great divide between nature and culture simply does not exist. For the Asmat of Papua New Guinea, for instance, some 'animals' are undeniably part of the 'human' family, whilst members of the neighbouring tribe come in to the category of foodstuff! I am quite convinced that the Asmat are mistaken. The problem is that I can only prove to them that they are mistaken from within my own culture (the same applies to them, always assuming that they are interested in 'converting' me to the Asmat *Weltanschauung*). Does that give me the right to force my convictions on them?

In my view, de-growth, in the sense that it provides the philosophical foundations for a project for an autonomous society, is probably not a humanism because it is based upon a critique of development, growth, progress, technology and, ultimately, modernity and because it implies a break with Western centralism. It is no coincidence that

most of those who inspired de-growth (Illich, Ellul, but
also Claude Lévi-Strauss, Robert Jaulin, Marshall Sahlins
and many others) denounce Western humanism.

The triumph of the imaginary of globalization, which is
a paroxysmal form of modernity, permitted and permits
an extraordinary attempt to delegitimate even the most
moderate relativist discourse. Along with human rights,
democracy and, of course, economics (thanks to the
market), cultural invariants are everywhere and are no
longer open to question. Western ethnocentrism, in the
form of the arrogant apotheosis of the market, is making
a comeback. Even anthropologists, who, as Lévi-Strauss
used to say, have a vocation for relativism, have shown
the white flag.[3]

The most recent attacks on relativism, now known as
'communitarianism', serve to mask 'especially since September 11', writes Annamaria Rivera (2005: 60), 'hege-
monic claims which frustrate earlier and painstaking
attempts to pursue translation policies that promote
mutual inter-communal and inter-cultural recognition'.
This 'universalist fanaticism' (Marta 2005) is amply demonstrated by recent statements from ideologists and politicians, including the Pope himself.[4]

As early as August 2000, a group of theologians under
the leadership of the then Cardinal Ratzinger (the future
Benedict XVI) was attacking the ideology of inter-faith
dialogue in the statement *Dominus Jesus* on the grounds
that it was an expression of 'relativist dogma'. The text
calls upon the Catholic Church to undertake a new mission
to evangelize other religious traditions because 'the full-
ness of the truth' can only be found in the Catholic Church.

---

[3] See, for instance, Françoise Héritier's denunciation of cultural relativism (Héritier 2007).
[4] After the attacks on the World Trade Center, the Italian journalist
Angelo Panebianco wrote, symptomatically, that: 'If the war on terror
lasts for years, we will have to take up arms to neutralize . . . the main
Western ally of Bin Laden and his consorts, or their most precious "fifth
column", namely cultural relativism' (cited Rivera 2005: 66).

This dogmatic stance destroyed the cross-cultural initiatives of Vatican II and the admirable work of the Indian-Catalan theological Raimon Panikkar, who has devoted his whole life to developing a matrix for inter-faith and inter-cultural dialogue. This universalist fanaticism is rightly denounced by Franco Cardini:

> We are faced with the systematic construction of a new totalitarianism that demonizes as 'relativist' any form of life and thought that differs from that imposed by the dominant paradigm and which claims to have a monopoly on the quest for the good and this earth by expelling any other form of thought or religious, civil and social vision because it is 'barbaric' or 'tyrannical'.[5] According to the Iranian Maryam Namzie, relativism is 'the fascism of our day' because it 'legitimates and fuels barbarism'.
> It asserts that the rights of individuals depend upon their nationality, their religions and their culture. . . . The supporters of cultural relativism state that we must respect culture and religion, even when they are despicable. . . . The defenders of cultural relativism have no qualms about saying that universal rights are a Western concept. . . . They are the defenders of the holocaust of our age.[6]

When we are faced with this ethnocentric universalist delusion, it is helpful to recall the recommendations of Melville J. Herskovits, who was one of America's greatest anthropologists. Addressing the UN Commission responsible for drafting the universal declaration of human rights[7]

---

[5] 'Il pensiero vuoto dei "necons" italiani', *L'Unità*, 25 August 2005, cited Rivera (2005: 69).

[6] In the same vein, Wassyla Tamzali vehemently exhorts us to 'wring the neck of the cultural relativism that is, strangely enough, even flourishing in the ranks of the intellectual left' (Namzie and Tamzali both cited Rivera 2005: 90).

[7] It was, it appears, General de Gaulle who convinced René Cassin, the French lawyer who drafted the declaration, that the term 'international' should be replaced by universal.

in his capacity as a member of the executive board of the American Anthropological Association in 1947, he made a preventive critique of universalism (that of universalist ideology, and not of the idea of universality). He argued that any attempt to formulate postulates derived from one culture's convictions or moral code made it more difficult to apply any declaration of human rights to humanity as a whole (cited Rivera 2005: 90). At the time, Herskovits' warnings and his demand for universality and plurality to be articulated went unheeded because of the fear that it might lead to a relativization of 'Nazi culture'. Islamism is the new spectre, and it is being used to justify the same refusal to contextualize human rights and to instrumentalize the legitimate demands of the women who are forced to live under *sharia* law.

Perhaps we should, in a word, be thinking about replacing the universalist dream, cleansed of its terrorist or totalitarian overtones – including the imperialism of growth – with the need to recognize what the Creole writer Raphaël Confiant calls 'diversality' or a 'pluriversalism' that is by definition relativist, or in other words a real 'democracy of cultures'. That is why the de-growth project is not a turnkey model, but a source of diversity.

Having said that, we must make it quite clear that this conception of de-growth is by no means an anti-humanism or an anti-universalism. Between the extremes of treating animals and things like people (as animists would) and treating people as things, as the modern techo-economy does, there is room for a respect for things, beings and people. Perhaps we could speak of an a-humanism, in the sense that I speak of a-growth. This certainly does not imply a rejection of all axiology, as my friend Michel Dias (2006) seems to think. On the contrary. It is not for nothing that the first 'R' in the virtuous circle that leads to de-growth is 're-evaluate'. The values we need (altruism, conviviality, respect for nature) are also the values that will allow us to begin a dialogue with other cultures without destroying them in the same way as the arrogant universalism of a dominant power, because we agree to recognize the relativity of our own beliefs. I do not, however, make this an absolute principle, and I do not feel that I have the right to prevent a Hindu from regarding killing a cow as murder, not that that will prevent me from enjoying a good steak.

The critique of modernity does not imply that we must simply reject it; it means, rather, that we have to transcend it. We have to denounce its bankruptcy and the triumphant heteronomy of the dictatorship of financial markets in the name of the emancipator project of the Enlightenment and the construction of an autonomous society.

Between the extremes of the blind or dogmatic anthropocentrism of Western modernity and the animist worship of nature, there is probably room for an eco-anthropocentrism (see Lanternari 2003). The very survival of humanity, and therefore of humanism in what we might call the true sense of that term, means that ecological concerns must be a central part of our social, political, cultural and spiritual preoccupation with human life. Recognizing that nature (animals, plants and everything else) has rights and fighting for 'eco-justice' and 'eco-morality' does not necessarily imply that we have to subscribe to the ecolatry of the new ecological cults or turn to the eco-feminist high priestesses of the syncretic neo-pagan and 'new age' cults that flourish all over the place to fill the emptiness in the soul of our aimless societies. Marxism is part of this tradition, which is why Hans Jonas writes: 'For Marx, the humanization of nature is a hypocritical euphemism for the total submission of nature to man so that he can exploit it completely in order to satisfy his own needs' (cited Lanternari 2003: 330).

I have argued that creating a de-growth society inevitably involves a re-enchantment of the world (see the conclusion to Latouche 2006a). But we have yet to agree what that means. The disenchantment of the modern world is at once simpler and more profound than Max Weber's analysis might suggest. It has less to do with the triumph of science and the disappearance of the gods than with the fantastic banalization of the things produced by the thermo-industrial system. In that sense, it really is a disenchantment and not just a 'demythologization'.[8] The use of vast quantities of the fossil energy that is freely supplied by nature both devalues human labour and authorizes the endless predation of natural 'wealth'. The result is a boundless artificial abundance that destroys all sense of wonder in the face of the gifts of the 'creator' and the creative abilities of human skill. The attempt to commercialize caribous in an Inuit community is a telling example (Godbout 2004: 420). The mayor of the village said to the government's spokesman:

> You know, we've been living with the caribou for a long time now, and I am not sure that we can do that to them. . . . The trouble is that introducing the caribou into the spatialized commodity circuit means cutting them off from their temporal network and the history of their relationship with the Inuit; we would have to turn them into objects, cut them into pieces and sell them, just as we do for the modern production process.

Artists object to this banal commodification because they play an irreplaceable role in building a serene de-growth society.

> Artists remind modern man that, whatever he does, he inevitably has to subscribe to some form of animism if he wants things to have a meaning. . . . Artists perhaps bear witness to the fact that animism is the only philosophy that

---

[8] We know that the success of Weber's formula is largely the result of a misunderstanding. The *Entzauberung* he talks about simply means that, in modernity, magical explanations are replaced by scientific explanations, rather as in Auguste Comte. Not all its effects are positive, but many of them are. Science is perfectly capable of enchanting a world in which there is no superstition. The banalization of 'wonders', on the other hand, is irremediable.

respects things and the environment; it is a philosophy that is adapted to the spirit of the gift that circulate in things, and modernity has cut us off from that. (Ibid.)

Animism or no animism, in a de-growth society, as Oscar Wilde puts it, 'All art is quite useless' . . . and therefore essential.

Bibliography

Aimé, Marco (2006), *Gli specchi di Gulliver*, Turin: Bollati.

Allende, Salvador Goosens (1973), *Speech Delivered by Dr Salvador Allende, President of the Republic of Chile, Before the General Assembly of the United Nations, 4 December 1972*, Washington, DC: Embassy of Chile.

Ariès, Paul (2005), *Décroissance ou barbarie*, Lyon: Golias.

Attac (2006), *Pauvreté et inégalité, ces créatures du néolibéralisme*, Paris: Mille et une nuits.

Attali, Jacques and Champain, Vincent (2005), 'Activité, emploi et recherche de l'emploi: changer de paradigme pour supprimer le chômage', Fondation Jean-Jaurès, no. 15, November.

Aubertin, Catherine and Vivien, Franck-Dominique, eds (2006), *Le Développement durable. Enjeux politiques, économiques et sociaux*, Paris: La Documentation française.

Aubin, Jean (2003), *Croissance: l'impossible nécessaire*, Le Theil: Planète bleue.

Bailly, Emmanuel (2006), 'Le Concept de l'Ecorégion ou comment restaurer le système immunitaire des regions', *Ligne d'horizon* 36, August–September.

Barras, Béatrice (2002), *Moutons rebelles: Ardelaine, la fibre du développement local*, Saint-Pierreville: Éditions Repas.

Baudrillard, Jean (2005), 'Nique ta mère!', *Libération*, 18 November.

Bauman, Zygmunt (1998a), *Globalization: The Human Consequences*, Cambridge: Polity.
—— (1998b), *Work, Consumerism and the New Poor*, Milton Keynes: Open University Press.
Baverez, Nicolas (2003), *La France qui tombe*, Paris: Perrin.
Belpomme, Dominique (2004), *Ces Maladies créées par l'homme*, Paris: Albin Michel.
—— (2007), *Avant qu'il ne soit trop tard*, Paris: Fayard.
Berlinguer, Enrico (1977), *Austerità. Occasione per trasformare l'Italia (Le conclusioni al convegno degli intellettualie (Roma, 15-1-77) e all'assemblea degli operai communisti (Milano, 30-1-77)*, Rome: Editori Riunti.
Berthouad, Arnauld (2005), *Une Philosophie de la cosommation. Agent économique et sujet moral*, Villeneuve d'Ascq: Presses universitaires du Septentrion.
Besset, Jean-Paul (2005), *Comment ne plus être progressiste . . . sans devenir réactionnaire*, Paris: Fayard
Besson-Girard, Jean-Claude (2005), *Decrescendo cantabile. Petit manuel pour une décroissance harmonique*, Lyon: Parangon.
Bevilacqua, Piero (2001), *Demetra a Clio: uomini e ambiente nella storia*, Rome: Donzelli.
—— (2006), *La Terra è finite. Breve storia dell' ambiente*, Bari: Laterz
Biehl, Janet, with Murray Bookchin (1998), *The Politics of Social Ecology: Libertarian Municipalism*, Montreal: Black Rose Books.
Blanc, Jérôme, ed. (2006), *Exclusion et liens financiers, Monnaies sociales, Rappport 2005–2006*, Paris: Economica.
Bloch, Ernst (1986) [1959], *The Principle of Hope*, trans. Neville Plaice, Stephen Plaice and Paul Knight, Cambridge MA, MIT Press, three vols.
Bologna, Gianfranco, ed. (2001), *Italia capace di futuro*, Bologna: WWF–EMI.
Bonaiuti, Mauro (2001), *La Teoria bioeconomica. La 'nuova economia' di Nicholas Georgescu-Roegen*, Rome: Ed. Carocci.
—— (2003), *Nicholas Geroescu-Roegen. Bioeconomia. Verso un'altra economia ecologicamente et socialmente sostenible*, Turin: Bollati Boriinghieri.
Bonesio, Luisa (2001), 'Une Réponse à la mondialisation', *Eléments* 100, March.

Bonora, Paola, 'Sistemi locali territoriali, transcalarità e nouve regole della democrazia del basso', in Anna Marsoon, ed., *Il Progetto della democrazia di territrio nella città metropolitana*, Florence: Alinea editrice.

Bookchin, Murray (1980), *Toward an Ecological Society*, Montreal: Black Rose Books.

—— (1982), *The Ecology of Freedom. The Emergence and Dissolution of Hierarchy* (revised edn), Montreal: Black Rose Books.

—— (2001), 'Interview with Murray Bookchin' by David Vanek, *Harbinger, A Journal of Social Ecology* 2(1).

Boulding, Kenneth E. (1996) [1966], 'The Economics of the Coming Spaceship Earth', in Victor D. Lippit, ed., *Radical Political Economy*, Armonk, NY: M.E. Sharpe.

Bové, José (2007), *Candidat rebelle*, Paris: Hachette Littératures.

Brillat-Savarin (1970) [1825], *The Philosopher in the Kitchen*, trans. Anne Drayton, Harmondsworth: Penguin.

Brown, Lester R. (2001), *Eco Economy: Building an Economy for the Earth*, London: Earthscan.

—— (2003), *Plan B: Rescuing a Planet under Stress and a Civilization in Trouble*, New York: Norton.

—— (2004), *Blueprint for a Better Planet*, Hendersonville, NC: Mother Earth News.

Brune, François (2004), *De L'Idéologie aujourd'hui*, Lyon: Parangon.

—— (2006), 'La Frugalité heureuse: une utopie', *Entropia* 1.

Bruni, Luigino (2002), 'L'Economia e i paradossi della felicita', in Pier Lugui Sacco and Stefano Zamagni, eds, *Complessita, relazionale e comparamento economica*, Bologna: Il Mulino.

Cacciari, Paolo (2006), *Pensare la descrescita. Sostenilità ed equità*, Rome/Naples: Cantieri Carta/Edizione Intra Moenia.

Caillé, Alain (2005), *Dé-penser l'économie. Contre le fatalisme*, Paris: La Découverte and MAUSS.

Canfin, Pascal (2006), *L'Économie verte expliquée à ceux qui n'y croient pas*, Paris: Les Petits Matins.

Castoriadis, Cornelius (1966), *La Montée de l'insignifiance: Les Carrefours du labyrinthe IV*, Paris: Seuil. (English edn: *Crossroads in the Labyrinth*, trans. Kate Soper and Martin Ryle, Cambridge, MA: MIT Press.

—— (2005), *Une Société à la derive*, Paris: Seuil.

Chanial, Philippe (2006), 'Une Fois commune: démocratie, don et éducation chez John Dewey, *Revue du MAUSS* 28.

Charbonneau, Bernard (1981), *Une Seconde Nature*, Pau: Bernard Charbonneau.

Charbonneau, Simon (n.d.), 'Résister à la croissance des grandes infrastructures de transport', Working document.

—— (2006), *Droit communautaire de l'environnement*, Paris: L'Harmattan, revised and expanded edn.

Cheynet, Vincent and Cheynet, Denis (2004), 'La Décroissance pour l'emploi', *La Décroissance* 3, July.

Cicolella, André and Benoît-Browaeys, Dorothée (2005), *Alertes santé*, Paris: Fayard.

Clément, Gilles and Jones, Louisa (2006), *Une Écologie humaniste*, Paris: Aubanel.

Clerc, Denis (2006), 'Peut-on faire l'économie de l'environnement?', *Cosmopolitiques* 13.

Cochet, Yves (2005), *Pétrole apocalypse*, Paris: Fayard.

—— and Sinaï, Agnès (2003), *Sauver la terre*, Paris: Fayard.

Dahl, Robert A. (1983), *Dilemmas of Pluralist Democracy: Autonomy vs Control*, New Haven: Yale University Press.

Decrop, Geneviève (2007), 'Redonner ses chances à l'utopie', *Utopia* 1.

Dias, Michel (2006), 'Un Idéalisme politique', *Entropia* 1.

Duclos, Denis (1997), 'Le Cosmocracie, nouvelle classe planétaire', *Le Monde diplomatique*, August.

Dumazedier, Joffre (1967) [1962], *Towards a Society of Leisure*, trans. Stewart E. McClean, New York: Free Press.

Dumouchel, Paul and Dupuy, Jean-Pierre (1979), *L'Enfer des choses*, Paris: Le Seuil.

Dupuy, Jean-Pierre (2002), *Pour un catastrophisme éclairé. Quand l'impossible est certain*, Paris: Le Seuil.

—— and Robert, Jean 1976), *La Trahison de l'opulence*, Paris: PUF.

Duval, Guillaume (2006), 'L'Impasse de la décroissance', *Cosmopolitiques* 13.

Ellul, Jacques (1998), *Métamorphoses du bourgeois*, Paris: La Table Ronde.

—— (2007), *Les Successeurs de Marx*, Paris: La Table Ronde.

Esteva, Gustavo (2004), *Celebration of Zapatismo*, Penang: Multiversity and Citizens' International.

—— and Prakash, M.S. (1998), *Grassroots Postmodernism: Remaking the Soil of Cultures*, London: Zed Books.

Flahaut, François (2005), *Le Paradoxe de Robinson. Capitalisme et société*, Paris: Mille et une nuits.

Flipo, Fabrice (2007), *Justice, nature et liberté. Les enjeux de la crise écologique*. Lyon: Parangon.

Fotopoulos, Takis (2001), *Vers une démocratie générale. Une démocratie directe, économique, écologique et sociale*, Paris: Le Seuil.

Galbraith, John Kenneth (1967), *The New Industrial State*, New York: Houghton-Mifflin.

Georgescu-Roegen, Nicholas (1971), *The Entropy Law and the Economic Process*, Cambridge, MA: Harvard University Press.

—— (1994), *La Décroissance: entropie, écologie, économie*, intro. and trans. Jacques Grinevald and Ivo Rens, Paris: Sang de la terre.

Gesualdi, Francesco (2005), *Sobrietà. Dallo spreco di pocji ai diretti per tutti*, Milan: Feltrinelli.

Gevaert, Pierre (2005), *Alerte aux vivants et à ceux qui veulent le reste*, Commarque: Ruralis.

Godbout, Jacques (2004), 'Les Conditions sociales de la création en art et en sciences', *Revue du MAUSS, 24, Une Théorie sociologique générale est-elle pensable?*

Gorz, André (1977), *Ecologie et liberté*, Paris: Galilée.

—— (1989) [1988], *Critique of Economic Reason*, trans. Gillian Handyside and Chris Turner, London: Verso.

—— (1994) [1991], *Capitalism, Socialism, Ecology*, trans. Chris Turner, London: Verso.

Grandstedt, Ingmar (2006), *Peut-on sortir de la folle concurrence? Petit manifeste à l'intention de ceux qui en ont assez*, Paris: La Ligne d'horizon.

Gras, Alain (2003), *Fragilité de la puissance*, Paris: Fayard.

—— (2006), 'Internet demande de la sueur', *La Décroissance* 35, December.

Grinevald, Jacques (2006), 'Histoire d'un mot. Sur l'origine de l'emploi du mot décroissance,' *Entropia* 1.

Guibert, Bernard and Latouche, Serge, eds. (2006), *Antiproductivisme, altermondialisme, décroissance*, Lyon: Parangon.

Harribery, Jean-Marie (2004), 'Développement durable: le grand écart', *L'Humanité*, 25 June.

Héritier, Françoise (2007), 'La Femme comme question politique', *Le Soir* (Brussels), 2 May.

Hoogendijk, Willem (1991), *The Economic Revolution. Towards a Sustainable Future by Freeing the Economy from Money-Making*, Utrecht: International Books.

—— (2003), 'Let's Regionalise the Economy – and Cure Ourselves of a Host of Ills,' trans. Nigel Harle, Utrecht: Stichting Aarde.

—— (2005), *Let's Stop Tsunamis*, Utrecht: Earth Foundation.

Hulot, Nicolas (2006), *Pour un pacte écologique*, Paris: Calmann-Lévy.

Illich, Ivan (1971), *Deschooling Society*, London: Calder and Boyars.

—— (1972), *Tools for Conviviality*, London: Calder and Boyars.

—— (1973), *Education without Schools*, ed. Peter Buchan, with contributions from Ivan Illich, London: Souvenir Press.

—— (1974), *Energy and Equity*, London: Calder and Boyars.

—— (1977), *Limits to Medicine. Medical Nemesis: The Expropriation of Health*, Harmondsworth: Penguin.

—— (1983), *Gender*, London: Marion Boyars.

Jacob, Jean (2006), *L'Altermondialisation. Aspects méconnus d'une nébuleuse*, Paris: Berg International.

Jacquart, Albert (1998), *L'Equation du nénuphar*, Paris: Calmann-Lévy.

Jacquiau, Christian (2006), *Les Coulisses du commerce équitable*, Paris: Mille et une nuits.

Jonas, Hans (1984) [1979], *The Imperative of Responsibility: In Search of an Ethics for the Technological Age*, trans. Hans Jonas with the collaboration of David Herr, Chicago: University of Chicago Press.

Jouvenel, Bertrand de (2002) [1968], *Arcadie. Essai sur le mieux vivre*, Paris: Gallimard.

Kempf, Hervé (2007), *Comment les riches détruisent la planète*, Paris: Le Seuil.

Kessous, Djémil (2006), *La Révolution moderne* (self-published).

Kurz, Robert (2006), *Critique de la démocratie balistique*, Paris: Mille et une nuits.

Lafargue, Paul (1907), *The Right to be Lazy, and Other Studies*, trans. C.H. Kerr, Chicago: Charles H. Kerr & Co.

Langlois, Bernard (2006), 'Bloc-notes', *Politis*, 14 December.

Lanternari, Victor (2003), *Ecoantropologia. Dall'ingerenza sociologica all svolta etico-culturale*, Baris: Edizionie Dedalo.

Latouche, Serge (1998), *L'Autre Afrique. Entre don et marché*, Paris: Albin Michel.

—— (2001), 'En finir une fois pour toute avec le développement', *Le Monde diplomatique*, May.

—— (2003a), *Justice sans limites. Le Défi de l'éthique dans une économie mondialisée*, Paris: Fayard.

—— (2003b), 'Pour une société de décroissance', *Le Monde diplomatique*, November.

—— (2003c), 'Il faur jeter le bébé plutôt que l'eau de bain', IUED, *Nouveaux cahier*, no. 14: *Brouillons pur l'avenir, contributions au débat sur les alternatives, avec ma réponse à Christian Coméliau.*

—— (2003d), 'La Décroissance comme prélable et non comme obstacle à une société conviviale', unpublished conference paper, Lyon.

—— (2004a), *Survivre au développement. De la décolonisation de l'imaginaire économique à la construction d'une société alternative*, Paris: Mille et une nuits.

—— (2004b), 'Antiproductivisme, décroissance, développement dirable et post-développement', La Tourette, Centre Thomas More, February.

—— (2004c), 'Objectif décroissance: la croissance en question', *Campagnes solidaires* 182, February.

—— (2004d), 'Pédagogie des catastrophes', *La Décroissance* 1, March.

—— (2004e), 'La Décroissance, pourquoi?' *Vert Contact* 709, April.

—— (2004f), 'Contre l'éthnocentrisme du développement. Et la croissance sauvera le Sud . . . .', *Le Monde diplomatique*, November.

—— (2005a), *L'Invention de l'économie*, Paris: Fayard.

—— (2005b), 'À Foi irrationelle dans le progress balaie toute objection' (interview), *CIO Stratégie et technologie*, March.

—— (2005c), 'Sortir de l'impasse de "l'effet rebond"', *Silence* 322, April.

—— (2005d), 'Pour une renaissance du local', *L'Ecologiste* 14, April–May.

—— (2005e), 'Le Défi de la décroissance', *Espace de liberté* (Brussels) 331, May.

—— (2005f), 'La Décroissance comme condition d'une société conviviale', *Cahiers Jacques Ellul* 3.

—— (2005g), 'Relocaliser l'économie', *La Décroissance* 28, September.

—— (2005h), 'Entretien sur la décroissance', *La Dynamo* 37, September.

—— (2005i), 'La Déraison de la croissance', *À Bâbord* 11, October–November.

—— (2005j), 'Écofascisme ou écodémocratie', *Le Monde diplomatique*, November.

—— (2005k), 'Vivre simplement pour que d'autres, simplement, puissent vivre', (interview), *Les Concentrés* (Brussels), November–December.

—— (2005l), 'Politique de décroissance: vivre localement', *Nature et progress* 555, November–December.

—— (2006a), *Le Pari de la décroissance*, Paris: Fayard.

—— (2006b), 'Penser une société de décroissance. Entretien avec Emmanuelle Martin', *Alliance pour une Europe des consciences* 7.

—— (2006c), 'La Decrescità', in Giovanna Ricoveri, ed., *Capitalism, natura, socialismo*, Milan: Jaca Book.

—— (2006d), 'La Déraison de la croissance', *L'Alpe* (revue du Musée dauphinoise) 32.

—— (2006e), 'Faut-il avoir peur d'abandonner la course à la croissance?' (interview), *Alternatives non-violentes* 138, March.

—— (2006f), 'Entretien', *Fibriles* (Liège) 6, Spring.

—— (2006g), 'Décroissance', in Sylvie Mesure and Patrick Savidan, eds, *Le Dictionnaire des sciences humaines*, Paris: PUF.

Lebow, Victor (1955), 'Price Competition in 1955', *Journal of Retailing* XXI(5), Spring.

Leclair, Bertrand (1998), *L'Industrie de la consolation. La Littérature face au cerveau global*, Paris: Verticales.

Lefebvre, Henri (1991–2005) [1968], *Critique of Everyday Life*, trans. John Moore, London: Verso, three vols.

Lietaer, Bernard (2006), 'Des Monnaies pour les communauté et les regions biogéographiques: un outil décisif pour la redynamisation régionale au XXIe siècle', in Jérôme Blanc, ed., *Exclusion et liens financiers. Monnaies sociales. Rapport 2005–2006*, Paris: Economica.

Ligne d'Horizon (2002), *Défaire de développement, refaire le monde (Actes du Colloque à l'UNESCO)*, Lyon: Parangon.

Lipotevsky, Gilles (2006), *Le Bonheur paradoxal, essai sur la société d'hyperconsommation*, Paris: Gallimard.

Lord-Nicholson, David (2006), 'The Numbers Game', *The Ecologist*, 22 September.

Lulek, Michel (2003), *Scions . . . travaillait autrement? Ambiance boi, l'aventure d'un collectif autogéré*, Saint-Pierreville: Éditions Repas.

Magnaghi, Alberto (2003), *Le Projet local*, Sprimont: Mardaga.

Marson, Anna, ed. (2006), *Il Progetto di territorio nella città metropolitana*, Florence: Alinea editrice.

Mansholt, Sico (1974), *La Crise*, Paris: Stock.

Maris, Bernard (2006), *Antimanuel d'économie. Tome 2: Les Cigales*, Paris: Bréal.

Marta, Claudio (2005), *Relzioni interetniche. Prospettive antropologiche*, Naples: Guida.

Martin, Hervé-René (2007), *Eloge de la simplicité volontaire*, Paris: Flammarion.

Martin, Douglas (2006), 'Murray Bookchin, 85, Writer, Activist and Ecological Theorist Dies', *New York Times*, 7 August.

Martinez Alier, Joan (2004), 'Che cos'è l'economic ecologica', in Andrea Masullo, ed., *Del mit della crecsita al nuvo umanesimo. Verso un nuovo modello di sviluppo sostenibile*, Grottaminigarda: Delta 3 Edizioni.

—— and Naredo, J.M. (1982), 'A Marxist Precursor to Energy Economics: Podolonsky', *Journal of Peasant Studies 9*.

Masullo, Andrea (1998), *Il pianeta di tutti. Vivere nei limiti perchè la terra abbia un futuro*, Bologna. EMI.

——, ed. (2004), *Dal mito della crescita al nuovo unamensimo. Verso un nuovo modello di svilluppo sostenibile*, Grottaminarda: Delta 3 Edizioni.

Meadows, Donella H., Randers, Jorgen and Behrens, W. (1972), *The Limits to Growth. A Report for the Club of Rome's Project on the Predicament of Mankind*, New York: Universe Books.

—— (1992), *Beyond the Limits to Growth. An Update*, Boston: Chelsea Green.

—— (2004), *Limits to Growth. The 30 Year Update*, Boston: Chelsea Green.

Méda, Dominique (1995), *Le Travail, une valeur en voie de disparition*, Paris: Alto-Aubier.

—— (2001), 'Notes pour en finir vraiment avec la fin du travail', *Revue du MAUSS*, 18.

Meyer, François (1954), *Problématique de l'évolution*, Paris: PUF.

—— (1974), *La Surchauffe de la croissance*, Paris: Fayard.

Mill, John Stuart (2004) [1848], *Principles of Political Economy*, Amherst, NY: Prometheus Books.

Monestier, Jean (2007a), 'Décroissance et travail', *Entropia* 2.

—— (2007b), 'La Grande Illusion des aéroports régionaux', *Fil du Confluent* 14, April–May.

Mothé, Daniel (1977), *L'Utopie del tempo libero*, Paris: Esprit.

Mühlstein, Philippe (2005), 'Les Ravages du movement perpetuel', *Le Monde diplomatique*, January.

Mumford, Stephen D. (1996), *The Life and Death of NSSM 200: How the Destruction of Political Will Doomed a US Population Policy*, Research Triangle Park, NC: Center for Research on Population and Security.

Napoleoni, Claudio (1990), *Cercare ancora. Lettera sulla laicità e ultimi scritti*, Rome: Editori Riunit.

Narboni, Camilla (2006), *Sulla incuria della cose: considerazioni filosfiche sui rifiuti e sul mondo saccaheggiato*, Pavia: University of Pavia.

Nicolino, Fabrice and Veillerette, François (2007), *Pesticides, revelations sur un scandale français*, Paris: Fayard.

Pallante, Maurizio (2005), *La Descrecita felice. La quantittà della vita no dipende dal PIL*, Rome: Editori Riuniti.

Panikkar, Raimon (2007), *Pour un pluriversalisme*, Lyon: Parangon.

Paquot, Thierry (2005), *Éloge du luxe. De l'Utilité de l'inutile*, Paris: Bourin éditeur.

—— (2006), *Terre Urbaine. Cinq défis pour le devenir urbain de la planète*, Paris: La Découverte.

—— (2007a), *Petit manifeste pour une écologie existentielle*, Paris: Bourin éditeur.

—— (2007b), *Utopie et utopistes*, Paris: La Découverte.

Partant, François (2002), *Que la crise s'aggrave*, with a preface by José Bové and an afterword by Serge Latouche, Lyon: Parangon.

Pasolini, Pier Paolo (2005), *Scritti corsari*, Milan: Garzanti Libri.

Perrot, Marie-Dominique, DuPasquier, Jean-Noël, Joye, Dominique, Leresche, Jean-Philippe and Rist, Gilbert, eds (2006), *Ordres et désordres de l'esprit gestionnaire*, Luzern: Éditions réalités sociales.

Petrini, Carlo (2006), 'Militants de la gastronomie', *Le Monde diplomatique*, July.

Prat, Jean-Louis (2007), *Introduction à Castoriadis*, Paris: La Découverte.

Rahnema, Majid (2003), *Quand la misère chasse la pauvreté*, Paris: Fayard/Actes Sud.

Ramaux, Christophe (2006), *Emploi: éloge de la stabilité. L'État social contre la flexicurité*, Paris: Mille et une nuits.

Rasmussen, Derek (2004), 'The Priced versus the Priceless' (*www.cis.yale.edu/agrarianstudies/papers/10rasmussen.pdf*).

Revel, Bernard (2005), *Journal de la pluie et du beau temps*, Canet: Trabucaire.

Ridoux, Nicolas (2006), *La Décroissance pour tous*, Paris: La Découverte.

Rifkin, Jeremy (1995), *The End of Work: The Decline of the Global Labour Force and the Dawn of the Post-Market era*, New York: Putman.

Rist, Gilbert (2006), 'La Nouvelle Gestion publique peut-elle être social?', in Marie-Dominique Perrot, Jean-Noël DuPasquier, Dominique Joye, Jean-Philippe Leresche and Gilbert Rist, eds, *Ordres et désordres de l'esprit gestionnaire*, Luzern: Éditions réalités sociales.

Rivera, Annamaria (2005), *La Guerra dei simboli. Veli postcoloniali et retorich sull'alterità*, Bari: Edizioni Dedalo.

Robin, Jacques (1994), *Quand le travail quitte la société post-industrielle*, Paris: GRIT-éditeur.

Rotillon, Gilles (2006), 'L'Économie de l'environnement définit un espace de négotiation rationnel,' *Cosmopolitiques* 13.

Rougemont, Denis de (1977), *L'Avenir est notre affaire*, Paris: Stock.

Ruffolo, Giorgio (2006), 'Crescita e sviluppo: critica e prospettive', *Falconara/ Macerata* 8/9, November.

Sachs, Wolfgang, ed. (1992), *Development Dictionary: A Guide to Knowledge as Power*, London: Zed Books.

Sahlins, Marshall (1972), *Stone-Age Economics*, Chicago and New York: Aldine Atherton.

Sas, Eva (2006), 'Conversion écologique de l'économie: quel impact sur l'emploi?', *Cosmopolitiques* 13.

Singleton, Michael (2006), 'Le coût caché de la décroissance', *Entropia* 1.

Stern, Nicholas (2006), 'The Economics of Climate Change: Executive Summary' (*www.sternreview-or.-uk*).

Tanguy, Philippe (2007), 'Pauvreté et cohesion sociale en Mauritanie. Construction sociale et function d'une catégorie stigmatisante: la pauvreté', *Revue Maghreb-Machreck* 109.

Tarde, Gabriel (1980) [1896], *Fragment d'histoire future*: Geneva: Slatkine.

Tertrais, Jean-Pierre (2006), *Du Développment à la décroissance. De la nécessité de sortir de l'impasse suicidaire du capitalisme*, Paris: Éditions du Monde libertaire.

Testart, Jacques (2006), *Le Vélo, le mur et le citoyen. Que reste-t-il de la science?*, Paris: Belin.

Tévoédjrè, Albert (1979), *Poverty: Wealth of Mankind*, Amsterdam: Elsevier.

Tomkins, Richard (2006), 'Welcome to the Age of Less', *Financial Times*, 10 November.

Veblen, Thorstein (1970) [1899], *The Theory of the Leisure Class*, London: Unwin Books.

Traoré, Aminata (2002), *Le viol de l'imaginaire*, Paris: Actes Sud/Fayard.

Virilio Paul (1984), *L'Espace critique*, Paris: Galilée.

—— (1995), *La Vitesse de liberation*, Paris: Galilée.

Waal, Frans de (2005), *Our Inner Ape: The Best and Worst of Human Nature*, London: Granta

Wackernagel, Mathis (2005), 'Il nostro planeta si sta esaurendo', in Andrea Masullo, ed., *Economia e ambient. La Sfida del terzo millenio*, Bologna: EMI.

Wackernagel, Mathis, et al. (2002), 'Tracking the Ecological Overshoot of the Human Economy', *Proceedings of the National Academy of Science USA* 99(14).

Worm, Boris, et al. (2006), 'Impacts of Biodiversity Loss on Ocean Ecosystem Services', *Science*, November, vol. 314, pp. 787–90.

WWF, *Living Planet 2006* (*http://assets.panda.org/downloads/living_planet_report.pdf*).

Zanotelli, Alex (2006), *Avec ceux qui n'ont rien*, Paris: Flammarion.

Zin, Jean, 'Les Limites de la décroissance', *La Décroissance*, January.

Journals and reviews consulted

Cahier de l'IUED 14: 'Brouillons pour l'avenir: contributions au débat sur les alternatives', Paris/Geneva: PUF, 2003.

Campagnes solidaires (Mensuel de la confederation paysanne) 182, February 2004.

Cosmopolitiques 13, 2006: 'Peut-on faire l'économie de l'evironnement?'

La Décroissance. Le Journal de la joie de vivre, Casseurs de pub, 11, place Croix-Pâquet, 69001 Lyon.

L'Écologiste 8, October 2002; 14, October 2004; 20, September–November 2006.

Entropia (Lyon: Parangon) 1, November 2006: 'Décroissance et politique'; 2, March 2007: 'Travail et décroissance'.

Le Figaro, 24 March 2006.

Libération, 8 February 2002; 18 November 2005; 14 December 2006.

Ligne d'horizon 36, August–September 2006.

Le Monde, 22 November 1991; 2 April 1996; 24 April 1999; 16 February 2002; 19 June 2003; 14 February 2004; 11 April 2004; 12 April 2004; 16–17 June 2005; 30 July 2006.

Le Monde diplomatique, May 2001; July 2004; January 2005.

Le Nouvel Observateur, 12–18 June 1972.

Politis, 11 December 2003; 14 December 2006.

Revue du MAUSS 24, 'Une Théorie sociologique générale est-elle pensable', 2nd quarter 2004.

Science 280, February 2002: 'La Peur de la décroissance'; 302, October 2003: 'Alternative-Alternative-Non-violence'.

Vert Contact 709, April 2004.

Index